Complete Care Skills

Gerardine Power

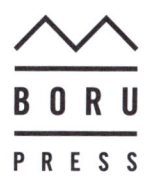

BORU PRESS

Boru Press Ltd.
The Farmyard
Birdhill
Co. Tipperary
www.borupress.ie

© Gerardine Power

ISBN 978 19160 1990 4

Design by Sarah McCoy
Print origination by Carole Lynch
Illustrations by Derry Dillon and Andriy Yankovskyy
Printed by GraphyCems Ltd, Spain

The paper used in this book is made from wood pulp of managed forests. For every tree felled, at least one tree is planted, thereby renewing natural resources.

All rights reserved. No part of this publication may be copied, reproduced or transmitted in any form or by any means without written permission of the publishers or else under the terms of any licence permitting limited copyright issued by the Irish Copyright Licensing Agency.

A CIP catalogue record for this book is available from the British Library.

For permission to reproduce photographs and artworks, the author and publisher gratefully acknowledge the following:

© Brendan McCormack 12. © Dr. Barman's 72. © Homecare Medical Supplies 65, 77, 92, 113, 114, 118, 119. © HSE 129, 130. © IASLT 93. © iStock 2, 11, 14, 17, 18, 19, 21, 22, 25, 29, 42, 71, 74, 75, 77, 81, 82, 92, 113, 118, 152. © Taylor & Francis Group 107. © World Health Organisation 51, 52, 54. © Zena Moore 132.

The author and publisher have made every effort to trace all copyright holders, but if any has been inadvertently overlooked we would be pleased to make the necessary arrangement at the first opportunity.

CONTENTS

1 Caring and Care Skills — 1

What is Care? — 2
Who Needs Care? — 2
Regulations and Standards — 3
What Qualities does a Carer Need? — 4
Elements of Holistic Care — 5
Adapting Care to the Individual — 14
Revision Questions — 15
Key Words and Phrases — 15

2 Working with Healthcare Professionals — 16

The Multidisciplinary Team — 16
Doctors — 17
Nurses — 17
Physiotherapists — 18
Occupational Therapists — 19
Dietitians and Nutritionists — 20
Speech and Language Therapists — 21
Orthoptists — 21
Podiatrists — 22
Psychiatrists — 22
Revision Questions — 23
Key Words and Phrases — 23

3 Good Communication — 24

Active Listening — 24
Verbal and Non-verbal Communication — 26
Personal Communication Tips — 30
Confidentiality — 32
Barriers to Communication — 32
Communicating Effectively with Clients with Hearing Problems — 32
Communicating with Others — 34
Revision Questions — 35
Key Words and Phrases — 35

4 Dignity and Respect — 36

Values in Action — 36
Empathy — 40
Promoting Independence — 41
Promoting a Positive Self-Image — 42
The Client's Personal Space — 43
Barriers — 43
Revision Questions — 44
Key Words and Phrases — 44

5 Hygiene — 45

The Client's Hygiene Needs — 46
The Carer and Hygiene Standards — 47
Hygiene Planning and Preparation — 47
Equipment — 58
Types of Assistance — 60
Cultural Considerations — 66

Aftercare	66
Revision Questions	68
Key Words and Phrases	68

6 Grooming, Dressing and Sensory Needs 69

Use of Sensory Equipment	70
Grooming	71
Dressing	75
Revision Questions	78
Key Words and Phrases	78

7 Meeting Nutritional Needs 79

Nutrition	79
The Food Pyramid	80
Assisting a Client at Mealtimes	89
Special Dietary Requirements	93
Cultural Considerations	96
After Mealtime	96
Recording and Reporting	96
Revision Questions	97
Key Words and Phrases	97

8 Continence Promotion and Toileting 98

Identifying the Level of Assistance Needed	99
Toileting Aids	99
Incontinence	103
Dignity and Respect	105
Cultural Considerations	106

Recording and Reporting	106
Revision Questions	108
Key Words and Phrases	108

9 Helping with Mobility — 109

Assessing the Client's Mobility Needs	109
Safety	111
Assisting with Mobility	112
Practical Tips for Assisting with Mobility	121
Manual Handling Regulations	122
Falls Risks	123
After Helping the Client	125
Revision Questions	126
Key Words and Phrases	126

10 Preventing Pressure Sores — 127

What is a Pressure Sore?	127
How to Assess a Pressure Sore	129
Caring for a Person at Risk of Getting a Pressure Sore	130
Record and Report	133
Revision Questions	134
Key Words and Phrases	134

11 Cleanliness and Preventing the Spread of Infection — 135

Cleaning Care Equipment and the Environment	136
Safe Management of Linen	138
Safe Waste Management	141

Revision Questions	143
Key Words and Phrases	143

12 Social Activities — 144

The Benefits of Socialising/Engaging in Activities	145
Barriers to Engaging in Activities	147
Client's Consent	148
Encouraging Involvement in Activities	148
Types of Activity	149
Cultural Considerations	153
Fitting Activities into Your Daily Routine	153
Planning and Preparation	155
Safety	156
After the Activity	156
Revision Questions	157
Key Words and Phrases	157

13 Safety — 158

Legislation	158
Risk Management	159
Manual Handling	160
Slips and Trips in the Healthcare Setting	162
Responding to Challenging Behaviour	163
Staff Immunisation	166
Revision Questions	167
Key Words and Phrases	167

14 Reporting and Documentation — 168

- What Should You Report? — 168
- How Do You Report? — 169
- Accident Reporting — 170
- Client Documentation — 170
- Revision Questions — 174
- Key Words and Phrases — 174

15 End of Life Care — 175

- Loss and Grief — 177

Appendices — 179

- 1 Food Intake Chart — 179
- 2 Fluid Balance Chart (fluid intake and output) — 180
- 3 Waterlow Chart — 181
- 4 Turns Chart — 182
- 5 Observation Chart — 183
- 6 Mood Chart — 184
- 7 Falls Risk Assessment Chart — 185
- 8 ABC Chart — 186
- 9 Mini Nutritional Assessment — 187

References — 188

Bibliography — 192

Useful Websites — 193

Index — 196

CARING AND CARE SKILLS 01

People have always cared for each other. When we lived as hunter-gatherers we didn't abandon the weak and sick – we looked after the members of the group who needed help. Caring for each other gave us a better chance of survival, especially when we lived in groups, with each member contributing to the whole group. Since those early times, we have evolved to become hard-wired to care for each other.

To care for others well, we need certain skills. While you may not have these skills at the moment, you can acquire them. To work as a carer and to carry out care skills well, you must first have caring and compassionate qualities or abilities. In this chapter we shall explore what it means to be caring and will look at the different aspects of care.

IN THIS CHAPTER YOU WILL LEARN ABOUT:

- The meaning of care and caring
- Who needs care
- The different elements of holistic care – physical, emotional, psychological and spiritual
- The importance of the individual when delivering care
- Maslow's hierarchy of needs
- Activities of daily living
- Adapting care to the individual

WHAT IS CARE?

Care can be defined as providing a person with what they need for their health, welfare and safety. It involves recognising and being aware of needs that the individual themselves cannot manage or meet. It is essentially doing something for another person, and being aware of that person's needs. Caring helps individuals meet their need to be healthy, active and as independent as possible. It helps individuals with everyday living and supports an individual's quality of life, their aims and desires.

Task Write down examples of how you have been caring towards others.

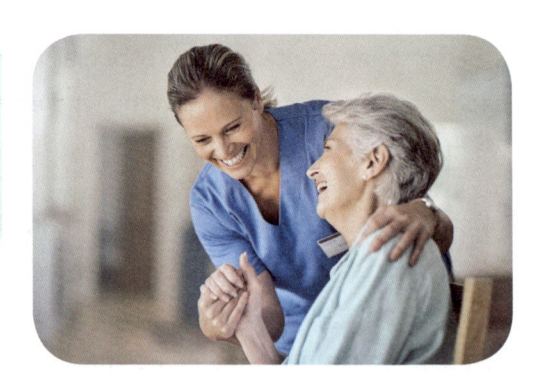

WHO NEEDS CARE?

At some point during our lifetime, each one of us will need care. As the English poet John Donne said, 'No man is an island'. We need other people and we all need to feel cared for.

Individuals who need care include:

- babies and children
- children with special/additional needs
- older people
- people near the end of their lives

- people who live with an intellectual disability
- people who live with mental health issues
- people who live with chronic health conditions
- people who live with a physical disability.

Care may be required at any time in life, from the moment we are born to the day we die – from the cradle to the grave.

Task Can you think of specific examples of people who need to be cared for?

REGULATIONS AND STANDARDS

Care Skills students will work in nursing homes looking after older people, in day care centres for the elderly, in hospitals, as home care helpers, with people living with physical or intellectual disabilities, and with clients who have a mental illness.

Many of these settings are inspected by HIQA (the Health Information and Quality Authority), an independent organisation which has the legal power and responsibility for improving the quality, safety and value of health and social care in Ireland (excluding mental health services).

HIQA is responsible for:

- setting standards
- monitoring and inspecting services
- providing guidance on health information
- carrying out health technology assessments.

The Health Act 2007 gives HIQA its powers over health and social care services in Ireland. Under this law, it is responsible for (among other things) developing national standards for health and social care services. The aim of these standards is to help drive improvements in the quality and safety of healthcare services in Ireland and to help the public, the people who use healthcare services and the people who provide them, understand what a high-quality, safe healthcare service looks like.

In particular, the standards:

- make sure that service providers are accountable to the public, service users and those who fund them

- help the people in charge of services identify what they are doing well, and where they need to improve

- help ensure that the quality and safety of services is the same no matter where people live in Ireland or what health service they use – no matter where the service is, it should be safe

- describe what should be in place for day-to-day services to be safe and effective (HIQA 2012).

WHAT QUALITIES DOES A CARER NEED?

It is useful to understand the difference between skills and qualities. A skill is an ability or expertise that can be learned through practice; a quality is a characteristic or trait that can be nurtured and developed. A carer needs many qualities to carry out their role.

Task Can you think of any qualities that would be useful?

CHAPTER 01: CARING AND CARE SKILLS

Qualities required in your role as carer:

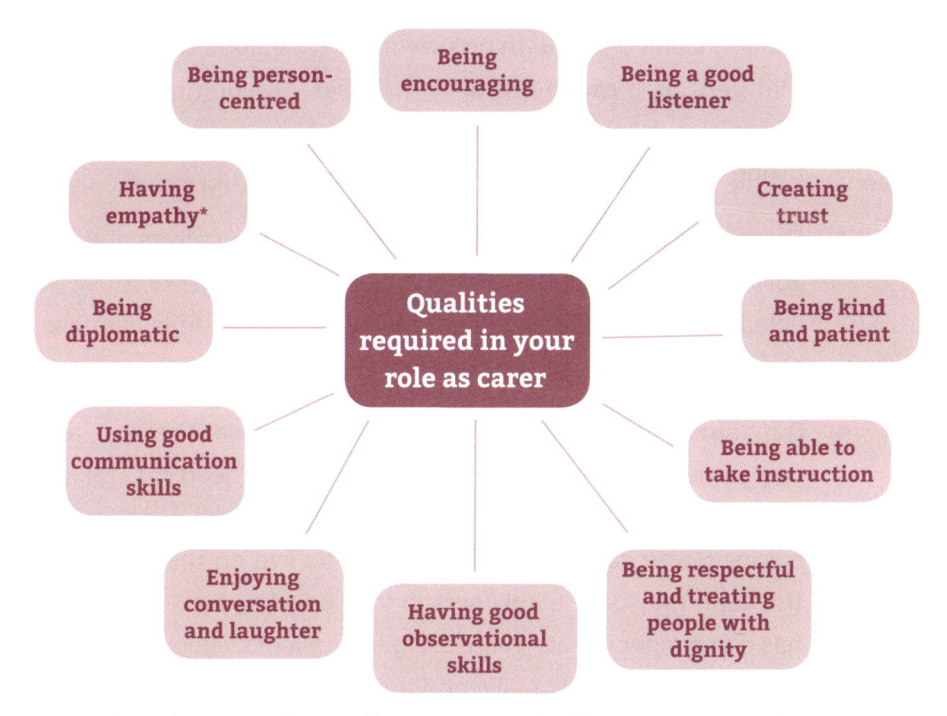

- Being person-centred
- Being encouraging
- Being a good listener
- Creating trust
- Being kind and patient
- Being able to take instruction
- Being respectful and treating people with dignity
- Having good observational skills
- Enjoying conversation and laughter
- Using good communication skills
- Being diplomatic
- Having empathy*

*__Empathy__ is having understanding or compassion for a person, an ability to put yourself in someone else's shoes. It is different from sympathy and from feeling sorry for someone.

ELEMENTS OF HOLISTIC CARE

Caring for a client involves looking after their physical, emotional, social, psychological and spiritual needs. We cannot provide for any of these needs in isolation. For example, when you are helping someone to wash, dress or eat, you are meeting their physical needs, but if you speak to them or smile at them while you're doing it, you can meet their emotional, social and psychological needs too. Whenever we help a client we should be attending to all or most of their needs at the same time.

+ Our **physical needs** include eating a balanced diet, taking regular exercise, following good hygiene practices and getting enough sleep – all the things we need for a good quality of life that gets us through our daily activities. Meeting our physical needs also means avoiding damaging habits such as smoking, taking drugs or drinking alcohol to excess.

- **Emotional needs** are met by understanding ourselves and our ability to cope with the challenges life can bring. We must be able to acknowledge and share feelings of anger, fear, sadness, stress, hope, love, joy and happiness in a productive way.

- Our **social needs** are fulfilled by our relationships and connections with other people in our world. We need to establish and maintain positive relationships with family, friends and carers. Some carers care for people who live on their own and the carer may be the only person they see every day. This carer has a very special role in ensuring their client's social needs are being met. A friendly smile and a chat are just as important as the person's physical needs.

- **Psychological needs** include our need for autonomy, competence and self-actualisation. Self-actualisation is personal growth and development throughout life; it means achieving your own full potential.

- **Spiritual needs** are the ways in which we establish peace and harmony in our lives. Many people achieve this through religion and by following religious rituals. Others, who don't believe in God or belong to any formal religion, may practise mindfulness or meditation, which helps them to gain an inner feeling of peace.

Maslow's Hierarchy of Needs

Maslow's hierarchy of needs is a motivational theory in psychology. It comprises a five-tier model of human needs. The basic principle of the theory is that the needs lower down in the hierarchy must be satisfied before we attend to needs higher up the scale.

Maslow's Hierarchy of Needs

Self-actualisation needs
achieving one's full potential, including creative activities
— Self-fulfillment needs

Esteem needs
prestige and feeling of accomplishment

Belongingness and love needs
intimate relationships, friends
— Psychological needs

Safety needs
security, safety

Physiological needs
food, water, warmth, rest
— Basic needs

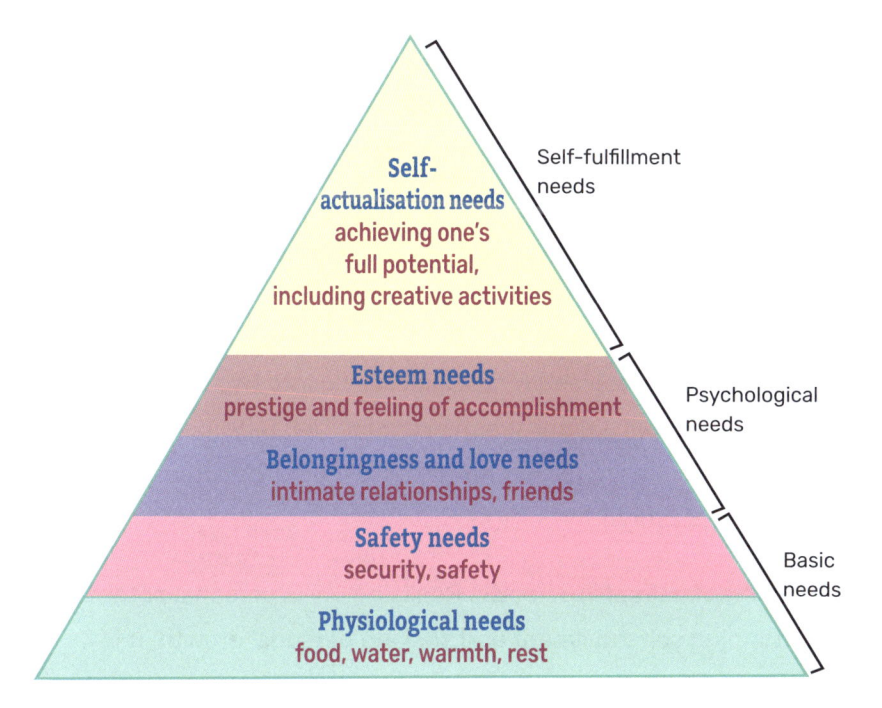

Maslow's idea is that everyone wants and is able to move up the hierarchy to the top level of self-actualisation. However, an individual's progress can be disrupted if they fail to meet lower-level needs. Negative life experiences, such as illness, divorce or job loss, can stall a person's progress, and they might slip backwards or fluctuate between levels of the hierarchy until life returns to normal. Not everyone will progress smoothly through the hierarchy – they may move back and forth between the different needs.

Our most basic need is for physical survival, so this is the first thing that motivates our behaviour. Once that level is fulfilled, the next level up is what motivates us, and so on.

1. **Physiological needs:** Biological requirements for human survival – air, food, drink, shelter, clothing, warmth, sex, sleep. Maslow considered physiological needs the most important because if they are not met, the other needs are irrelevant.

2. **Safety needs:** Protection from the elements, security, order, law, stability, freedom from fear.

3. **Belongingness and love needs:** Our social needs – friendship, intimacy, trust and acceptance, receiving and giving affection and love. This need also includes being part of a group (family, friends, work).

4. **Esteem needs:** Maslow classified these into two categories: (i) self-esteem – dignity, achievement, mastery, independence; and (ii) the desire for reputation or respect from others (e.g. status, prestige).

5. **Self-actualisation needs:** Realising one's personal potential, attaining self-fulfilment and seeking personal growth. It is a desire 'to become everything one is capable of becoming' (Maslow 1987:64).

In summary, human beings are motivated by a hierarchy of needs. The most basic needs must be satisfied before the subsequent sets of needs can be considered. It is important to remember this in the care setting and to ensure that the client's basic needs are always met. Speaking intelligently and respectfully to patients will demonstrate respect (esteem needs), while forming a bond with clients will satisfy their need for belonging.

The case study will help to explain the different aspects of care.

Case Study: Best Practice

It's your first day at work in a nursing home. You are asked to care for an 85-year-old woman, Annie, who has had a stroke and suffers from arthritis. What are her needs?

+ **Physical needs**

    – Annie might need help with an assisted wash (bed bath, shower/bath, bowl by bedside or wash at sink) and dressing (consider her choice of clothes, footwear, etc.).

    – Mobilising – does she need help with walking and, if so, what kind of help?

    – Toileting – does she need help going to the toilet, is she wearing incontinence wear, does she have a catheter?

    – Eating and drinking – what kind of food does Annie eat, what does she like, does she need assistance?

+ **Emotional**

    What kind of support does Annie get from her family, friends and community? Annie will want to feel loved, cared for and accepted. At all times treat Annie with respect and understanding. We all need to have our feelings and emotions respected.

    When you are washing Annie, treat her with respect. If she is upset or anxious, listen to her worries. Giving her explanations and choices will make her feel included in her care and worthwhile. If you treat her as an individual and show an interest in her, you will be tending to her emotional care.

✚ Social

Family and friends are part of our social life. If they and Annie wish, they should be included in Annie's care. They should be made welcome to visit. Other residents in the nursing home and the nursing home staff are also an important part of Annie's social life. Residents often eat together, sit together and have activities and social events planned for most days. Not everyone enjoys these group social activities, so find out what Annie likes doing. Offer her opportunities to take part in social occasions, but respect her wishes if she prefers to spend time on her own. While attending to Annie's physical care, e.g. helping her to wash, chat to her – you are part of Annie's social life too.

✚ Psychological needs

Annie must be included in her care and allowed to make decisions. She should be given choices and have her wishes respected. Don't forget that she is an individual. Every person is different and unique, so care should be given in an individual way rather than as part of a routine. Annie needs to be the person in control of her care; she needs to be as independent as possible. The carer must always treat her with empathy and respect.

When assisting Annie with sensitive procedures, treat her with respect and dignity. Encourage her to attend to her own needs if possible and take her wishes into account. She should be able to decide what help she needs. If we take away these choices, which is taking away her independence, this will have a psychological effect on Annie. She may feel depressed and helpless.

> **+ Spiritual needs**
>
> We often think of spiritual needs as religious needs. What are Annie's religious needs? Does she wish to attend mass, have a priest visit, etc.? We need to respect the wishes of the client if their beliefs are different from ours. There are other aspects of spiritual needs too. The need for meaning and purpose in life, the need to give and receive love and also the need for forgiveness, creativity and hope are fundamental to our well-being. Be aware of different religious needs as well as non-religious needs and facilitate the client in meeting their beliefs and rituals.

Person-centred Care

Person-centred care simply means that the person you are caring for is at the centre of all decisions. The needs of the person are more important than the needs of the services. All care should be planned and delivered around the person needing care. They should be looked at holistically and as an individual. It recognises what the patient feels, how they engage and participate in decisions about their care as well as the values that underpin the management of the healthcare system.

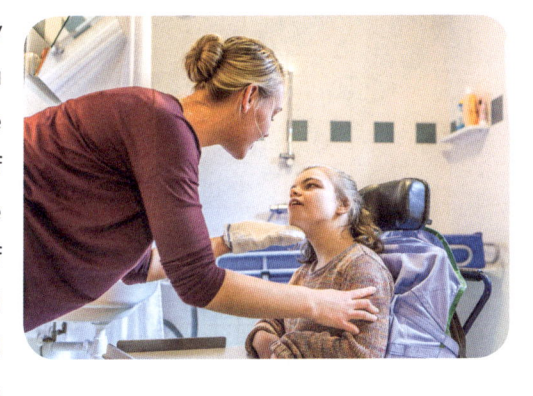

The World Health Organisation's (WHO) definition of health indicates that it is not only the physical needs of patients that need to be addressed but also their psychological, social, spiritual and environmental needs (WHO 1946).

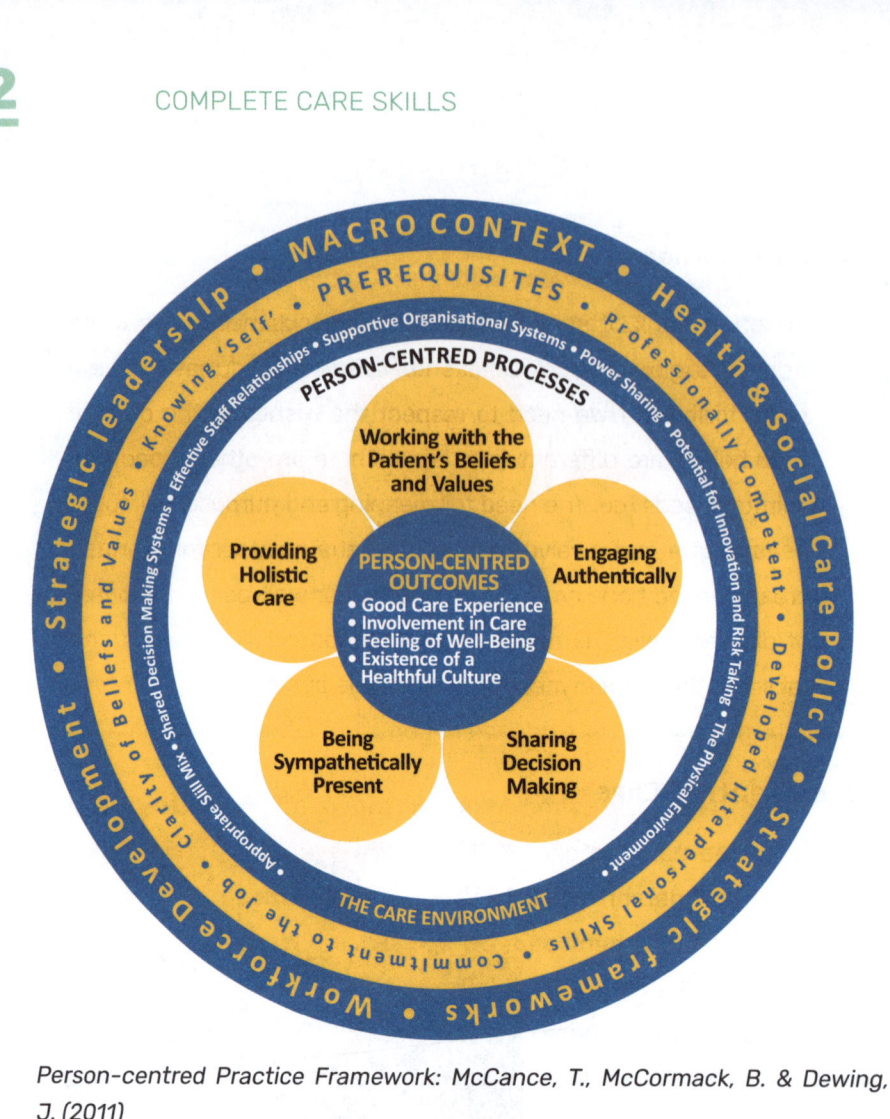

Person-centred Practice Framework: McCance, T., McCormack, B. & Dewing, J. (2011)

HIQA's National Standards for Safer Better Healthcare consists of eight themes: Theme 1 is about person-centred care and support, and it details how healthcare should respect the values and dignity of its clients and be responsive to their rights and needs. The wishes and needs of each individual should also be balanced with those of other clients. HIQA uses the Person-centred Practice Framework to describe a standard of care that ensures the client is at the centre of care delivery. Healthcare service providers should focus their work on the needs and preferences of clients rather than on what is convenient for the service provider (HIQA 2012).

Activities of Daily Living

Everyone carries out everyday activities that are essential to normal functioning. Roper, Logan and Tierney (2000) identified twelve daily activities that can be used to assess patients or care clients. A client's ability to perform these activities independently is analysed to see how their life may have changed due to illness or a change in their health. Assessment of activities of daily living (often abbreviated to ADL) identifies any client issues and creates a plan of action that will support and encourage independence in any area that may be difficult or impossible for the client to achieve on their own. The ADL scale assesses the client's independence and potential for independence on a continuum ranging from complete dependence to complete independence.

The goal for the carer is to maximise the independence of the client. It is also important to maintain the client's normal routine as far as possible. In many healthcare workplaces, the ADL model is used to plan care for the clients. Individual care plans are designed around the identified needs of the client. This helps determine what actions need to be taken and what ongoing support is required to compensate for any dependency. The assessment must be reviewed continuously to determine whether the plan is working and whether the client has any new needs due to a deterioration in their condition. If the client has new needs, care plans may have to be changed to meet them.

The ADLs are:

- Maintaining a safe environment
- Communication
- Breathing
- Eating and drinking
- Elimination
- Washing and dressing
- Controlling temperature
- Mobilisation

- Working and playing
- Expressing sexuality
- Sleeping
- Death and dying.

To provide effective care, all the client's needs must be met by: supporting them to meet those needs independently; providing the care directly; or a combination of the two.

ADAPTING CARE TO THE INDIVIDUAL

The care we deliver should never be the same for every client. It is important that we assess the needs of each client as an individual and provide the tailored care they require. We assess their needs by consulting the client's care plans, the handover report from the nurse-in-charge, and by looking at and talking to the client. This helps us to build a picture and plan the care needed for each individual.

For example, let's say you are caring for four clients in a nursing home. Client one may need a full bed bath, client two may need a shower, client three may only need an assisted wash and client four may not need any help. We adapt the care we give according to the needs of the client.

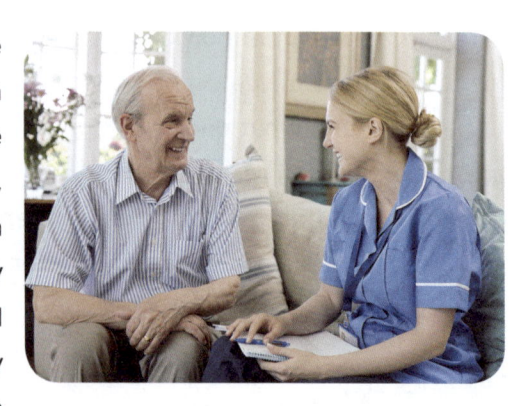

Exercise:

You are asked to look after a 20-year-old man, Jason. All you have been told is that he requires the use of a wheelchair following a car accident.

+ How will you find out how much help Jason is going to need?
+ What kind of social needs will Jason have?
+ How do you think you can help him to meet these needs?

Revision Questions:

1. What is care and what does it mean to be caring?
2. What different groups of people need care?
3. What are the needs in Maslow's hierarchy of needs?
4. List the activities of daily living (ADL).
5. What are the different elements of caring?

Key words/phrases:

Maslow's hierarchy of needs

person-centred care

activities of daily living (ADL)

person-centred care

HIQA (Health Information and Quality Authority)

WHO (World Health Organisation)

WORKING WITH HEALTHCARE PROFESSIONALS

02

IN THIS CHAPTER YOU WILL LEARN ABOUT WORKING WITH:

- Doctors
- Nurses
- Physiotherapists
- Occupational therapists
- Dietitians/nutritionists
- Speech and language therapists
- Orthoptists
- Podiatrists
- Psychiatrists

THE MULTIDISCIPLINARY TEAM

Healthcare assistants help clients with some or all of their activities of daily living. It is the duty of the care facility nurse to assess, plan, implement and evaluate the care required by the client. The primary role of the healthcare assistant is to assist the nurse in the implementation of this plan. In the care of your client, you will encounter a number of different healthcare professionals who have responsibility for their particular field of expertise but work as a multidisciplinary unit to care for the client. The healthcare team can include nurses, physiotherapists, occupational therapists, dietitians/nutritionists, speech and language therapists, orthoptists, podiatrists and psychiatrists.

DOCTORS

Doctors assume complete responsibility for a client's care. Acting in their best interest, the doctor establishes and maintains trust in the doctor/client relationship. Doctors' obligations of trust are contained in the codes of practice and codes of ethics of the medical profession, historically linked to the oath of Hippocrates. Doctors make diagnoses, are up-to-date on the most appropriate treatment, respond to clients' needs and take complete responsibility for the client's care. If more specialised care is required, the doctor will refer the client to a colleague or consultant. Other members of the medical team look to the doctor for leadership in designing and supervising the client's overall health care plan. Doctors support clients to make decisions about their own healthcare.

NURSES

Nurses care for people's emotional, psychological and physical needs. They aim to promote the health of the individual and are responsible for planning and implementing the complete nursing care of their patients. They assess nursing needs, draw up care plans, observe the effectiveness of care and modify the care plan accordingly. They administer medicine and injections and carry out routine procedures.

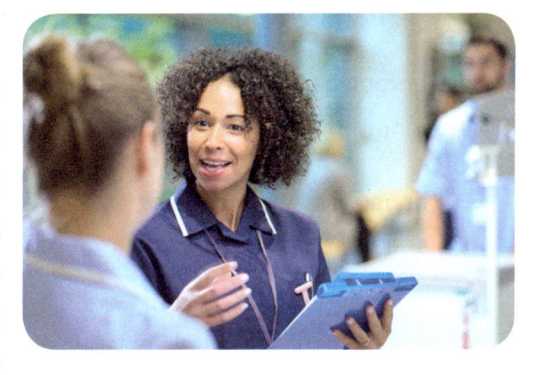

Nurses of any discipline might work in hospitals, community-based health centres or in patients' homes. Some concentrate on health promotion work, for instance helping patients regain or retain their independence, which allows them to continue living at home.

PHYSIOTHERAPISTS

Physiotherapists work with people with injuries to the musculoskeletal system. Functional movement is central to what it means to be healthy, and physiotherapy helps to restore movement and function when someone is affected by injury, illness or disability. It can also help to reduce the risk of injury or illness in the future.

Evidence has shown that physiotherapy can:

- help reduce the risk of falls and fractures
- maintain and improve functional ability, including gait
- promote mental health and well-being
- reduce length and cost of hospital stay
- improve continence.

Physiotherapy can be helpful for people of all ages with a wide range of health conditions, including problems affecting the:

- bones, joints and soft tissue – such as back pain, neck pain, shoulder pain and sports injuries
- brain or nervous system – such as movement problems resulting from a stroke, multiple sclerosis (MS) or Parkinson's disease
- heart and circulation – such as rehabilitation after a heart attack
- lungs and breathing – such as chronic obstructive pulmonary disease (COPD) and cystic fibrosis (ISCP).

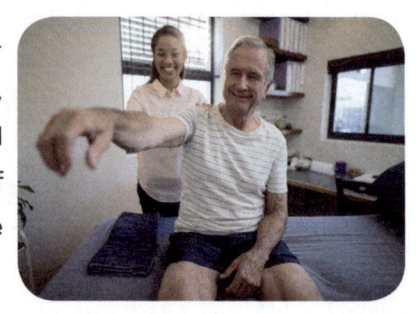

In addition, exercise improves cardio-respiratory function, muscle function, flexibility, participation in physical activity, and the functional ability of frail older adults. In some care settings there is a separate physiotherapy department, where you may be required to take the client. You might be involved in the physiotherapist's programme, helping to teach the client new adaptive skills or helping them with mobility or special exercises for which they need your support (HSE 2012a).

OCCUPATIONAL THERAPISTS

Occupational therapy is a client-centered health profession concerned with promoting health and well-being through occupation. The primary goal of occupational therapy is to enable people to participate in the activities of everyday life. The occupational therapist (OT) provides support to people whose health prevents them doing the things that matter to them – washing, dressing, getting to the shops, cooking, etc. They identify goals that can help the client maintain, regain, or improve independence by using different techniques, changing the environment and using new equipment. Occupational therapists work with people of all ages and can look at all aspects of daily life, from the home to the school or workplace (AOTI).

Occupational therapy:

+ promotes health and well-being through the use of occupation
+ helps reduce falls in older people who are at high risk of falling
+ improves physical and mental health, social well-being and life satisfaction
+ improves the quality of life, mood and health status of both clients and carers
+ improves functional mobility, self-care and home management activities

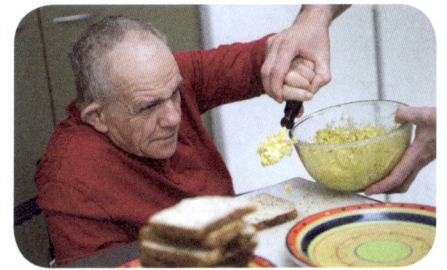

- improves the daily functioning of older people with dementia and their carer's sense of competence

- provides training in self-care activities to the older person using adaptive medical equipment and/or compensatory techniques if required.

It focuses on increasing or maintaining functional independence, social participation and quality of life, both from a preventive perspective and a treatment perspective (HSE 2012a).

There is a wide range of care aids available to help a client with daily living activities: see Assist Ireland (www.assistireland.ie) for information on daily living aids, mobility aids and assistive technology, as well as lists of suppliers of such equipment in Ireland. Care aids listed include ramps and stairlifts, hoists and slings, manual and powered wheelchairs, children's daily living equipment, showering and bathing equipment, and eating and drinking equipment. Assist Ireland has been developed by the Citizens Information Board in association with disability organisations, service providers and support agencies both in Ireland and abroad.

In some settings, the carer may have to take the client to a designated OT department. The client is unlikely to see the OT every day, and on days when the client doesn't see the OT, it's important that the carer continues to support the client to be independent. It may take more time, but the carer needs to continue with the techniques learned in therapy. The carer is supporting the role of the OT for the benefit of the client. The carers and OT work together, and good communication is important.

DIETITIANS AND NUTRITIONISTS

Nutrition is an important part of the management of chronic diseases, malnutrition and general abilities of the older person. It can help prevent many conditions and diseases and is a key component of quality of life.

The dietitian's role is to identify and assess malnutrition risk; implement suitable lifestyle changes; and draw up nutrition plans for the client, their family and staff.

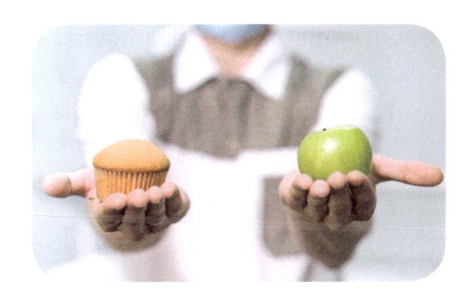

SPEECH AND LANGUAGE THERAPISTS

Speech and language therapists provide life-changing treatment, support and care for children and adults who have difficulties with communication, or with eating, drinking and swallowing. They help people who, for physical or psychological reasons, have problems speaking and communicating. Patients range from children whose speech is slow to develop to older people whose ability to speak has been impaired by illness or injury.

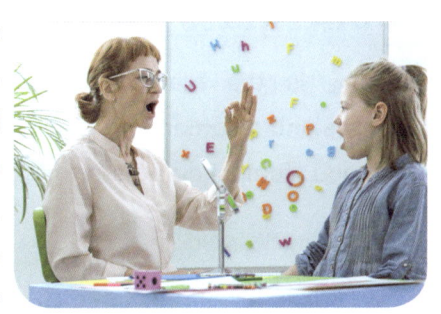

ORTHOPTISTS

Orthoptists investigate, diagnose and treat defects of binocular vision and abnormalities of eye movement. For example, they may deal with:

- misalignment of the eyes (strabismus or squint)
- double vision (diplopia)
- reduced vision (amblyopia)

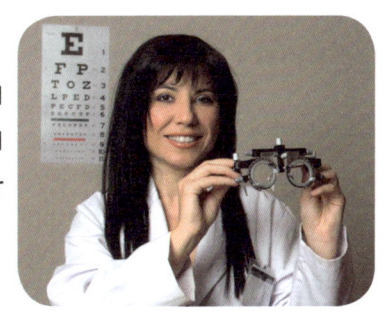

An orthoptist will, for example:

- assess the vision of babies and small children, including children with special needs
- help with the rehabilitation of patients who have suffered stroke or brain injuries
- diagnose and monitor long-term eye conditions such as glaucoma.

PODIATRISTS

Podiatry is the management of diseases and disorders of the lower limb and foot. Podiatrists might work on:

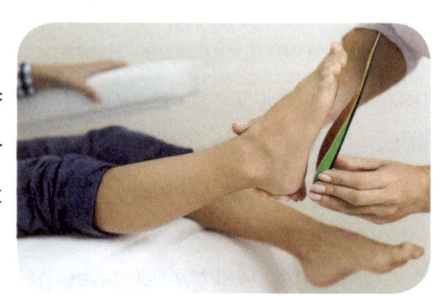

- helping children with lower limb pain or problems walking
- helping diabetes sufferers who may be at risk of amputation with circulation problems
- helping people with sports injuries and dancers whose long hours of rehearsing and performing put stress on their feet.

PSYCHIATRISTS

Psychiatry of old age (POA) provides specialist mental health services for older people and specifically for people who develop mental disorders over the age of 65 years. It responds to the needs of two groups of people:

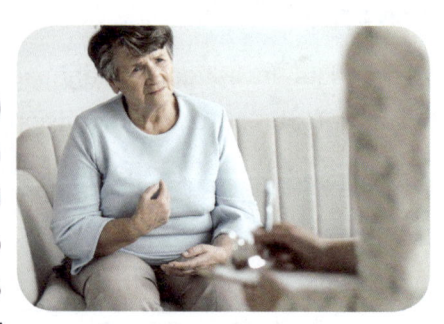

CHAPTER 02: WORKING WITH HEALTHCARE PROFESSIONALS

1. Older people (over 65) who develop functional psychiatric disorders such as depression.

2. Dementia sufferers with behavioural or psychological problems for which psychiatric intervention is required.

Specialist psychiatric services specifically for older people are required because:

+ Many people become mentally ill for the first time over the age of 65 years, partly because of losses, such as bereavement, and physical ill health, but also because of pathological changes in the brain – which are reflected in the dementias.

+ Changing demographic factors mean that more people are surviving to old age and, therefore, more people are at risk of developing dementia (HSE 2012a).

Revision Questions:

1. Name three healthcare professionals who might be involved in the care of your client.
2. Names two ways in which you would support each of these healthcare professionals.

Key words/phrases:

- nursing
- physiotherapy
- occupational therapy
- dietitian
- nutritionist
- speech and language therapist
- orthoptist
- podiatrist
- psychiatry of old age

GOOD COMMUNICATION 03

A great deal of information is passed every day from the client to the carer and from the carer to the client, so the carer must be a good communicator.

When talking about feelings or attitudes, communication is made up of 7% verbal communication (what we say), 38% vocal communication (how we say it) and 55% non-verbal communication (body language). (*Mehrabian, A. 1981*)

Communication involves both passing information to other people *and* receiving information from others. It is a two-way process (HSE Guidelines).

> **IN THIS CHAPTER YOU WILL LEARN ABOUT:**
>
> + Communication as a two-way process
> + Listening skills
> + Non-verbal communication
> + Effective communication
> + What we need to communicate
> + The importance of confidentiality
> + Barriers to communication
> + Communicating with the team

ACTIVE LISTENING

Listening can be passive or active. Listening to someone as background noise, without focusing on what the person is saying, is *passive* listening. Carers need to listen very attentively to their clients – this is *active* listening. Listening to a person actively helps promote their sense of worth because it will make them feel that what they have to say matters.

Communication is a two-way process. It is important to not only listen to but to hear the message. Time is needed for effective communication. A person who has difficulty speaking or hearing or who has difficulty processing or retaining information may require more time. Give communication as much time as is needed for everyone involved to communicate and understand the message.

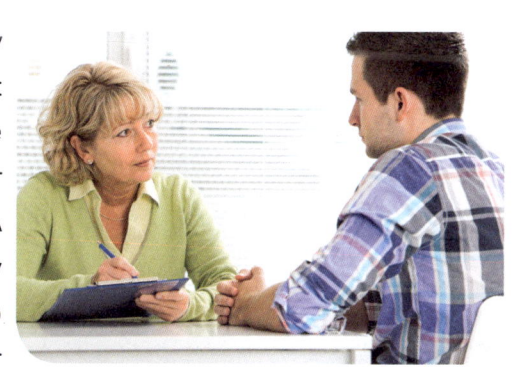

Listening skills are as important as speaking skills. When listening we should show interest in what the other person is saying. Allow them time to speak and don't interrupt. Make eye contact when they are speaking. Our body posture can be used to show that we are interested in what the other person is saying, for example by leaning forward slightly.

Sometimes it can be difficult to understand what another person is saying. Repeat what they have said and ask for clarification. People can sometimes forget what they have been told. If you are being told something important, for example instructions from your supervisor, write it down. Don't rely on memory.

> **Task**
>
> **Chinese Whispers.** Whisper a silly sentence to your neighbour. Get them to pass it on. Keep passing it on along the class. Ask the last person to say what they have just heard. Is it the same as the starting sentence?

VERBAL AND NON-VERBAL COMMUNICATION

Communication can be both verbal and non-verbal. Verbal communication uses words – it is spoken. Non-verbal communication involves all the other ways in which we pass information on to others, including our body language, facial expression and hand gestures. Sometimes we are aware that we are communicating in this way; at other times we are not. A teacher can easily tell which students in the classroom are interested in what they are saying, just by their body language and their facial expressions.

> **Task** Describe a student who looks as though they are interested in the class. Describe a student who looks as though they are not interested in the class.

Verbal Communication

Verbal communication is the words we use to communicate with others. For communication to take place, others must understand what we are saying. There are a number of ways of ensuring that we are understood.

- **Tone and pitch:** When we speak, our voice naturally goes up and down, louder and quieter, adding meaning to the words. Our tone should always be friendly when speaking to clients. Never shout at a client or use bad language.

- **Avoid jargon:** We often use medical language or abbreviations in care settings. The client may not be familiar with these. Use simple, clear language that the client will understand.

- **Speak clearly:** If we are giving instructions to the client, it should be given in clear and simple steps.

- **Language:** Sometimes we must care for clients who do not speak English, or for whom English is not their first language. It is important that information is provided in their own language. Some care settings may have access to a translator. Relatives and friends can also help with some translating, but you must be aware of confidentiality. You could learn some simple words and phrases in the client's language to help you deliver day-to-day care. Technology can help, or you could use a translating tool such as Google Translate. Visual signs and symbols can help a client to understand, e.g. a menu with pictures of food would be more helpful than one with just words.

- **Accents:** Some of us speak with a strong accent, which can be hard for people from a different region to understand. Be aware that if you have a strong accent you may need to speak more slowly and clearly.

- **Hearing impairment:** Be aware that the client may have a hearing deficit. Don't shout at a client who is hard of hearing. Instead speak slowly and clearly. If they are wearing a hearing aid, make sure that it is in place and switched on.

Non-verbal Communication

Non-verbal communication, such as gestures, facial expressions and appropriate touch, can be important when communicating with people who are experiencing communication difficulties. Gestures and facial expressions can be used to express an emotion, e.g. a thumbs-up can reassure a person that things are all right.

Our facial expressions normally reflect our words, our feelings and the situation we are in. If you went to the doctor for some important test results and she had a big smile on her, face you wouldn't expect her to say, 'I'm sorry, but the news is bad.' When we are caring for clients we should try to appear cheerful and smile at them. As we chat to them our expression will change to show empathy and interest in what they are saying.

- **Body language:** We can communicate a lot of information with our body language. Do you ever people-watch? Even though you cannot hear what they are saying, you can interpret the situation by their body language. If you tell a client with your hands on your hips that you are going to help them have a wash, they might think, 'Well, she means business – this will be quick.' Our body language should be non-threatening to the client, so adopt a neutral body stance and try not to invade their space. We all have a space around us – our personal space – that only certain people can enter. A carer has to enter this body space when delivering personal care. Be respectful when doing so, as it may make the client feel uncomfortable.

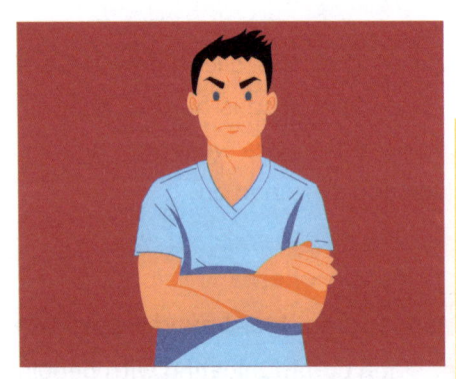

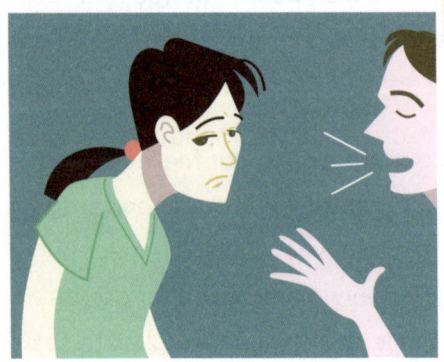

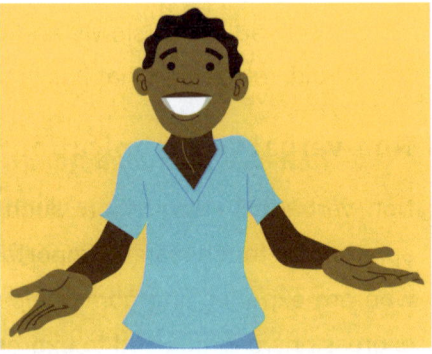

> **Task** What messages do you read/receive from the body language in these images?

- **Eye contact:** Making eye contact with the client when communicating shows that you are interested and that you can be trusted. But don't stare – this will make them feel uncomfortable. However, in some cases it may be appropriate to avoid eye contact, especially if a client is angry and upset, when direct eye contact may be seen as confrontational.

- **Touch:** Sometimes it is appropriate to communicate to the client without words. Holding the hand of an anxious person shows without words that you are there for them. Sometimes we don't have the words to make an upset person feel better, but touch can help. It is important to accurately read the body language of the client when holding their hand. If they stiffen and look uncomfortable, this may indicate that they don't want to have their hand held.

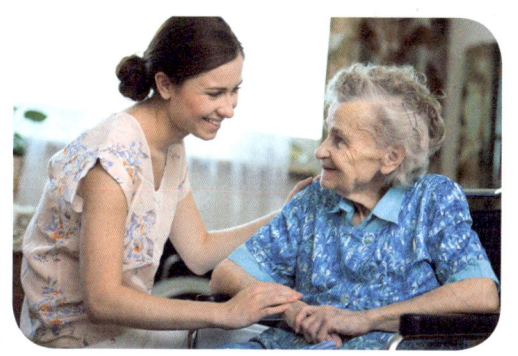

- **Non-verbal communication by the client:** It is possible to assess the needs of a client who cannot speak by looking at their body language and by careful observation. For example, a client in pain will show it on their face and they may be very restless. Carers are often the best at understanding a client's non-verbal communication as they know the client best.

- **Visual aids:** Drawings, diagrams or photographs are a useful tool in communicating information, especially with someone who is deaf or hard of hearing, or someone with an intellectual disability or a brain injury. They can point at a picture to express their needs.

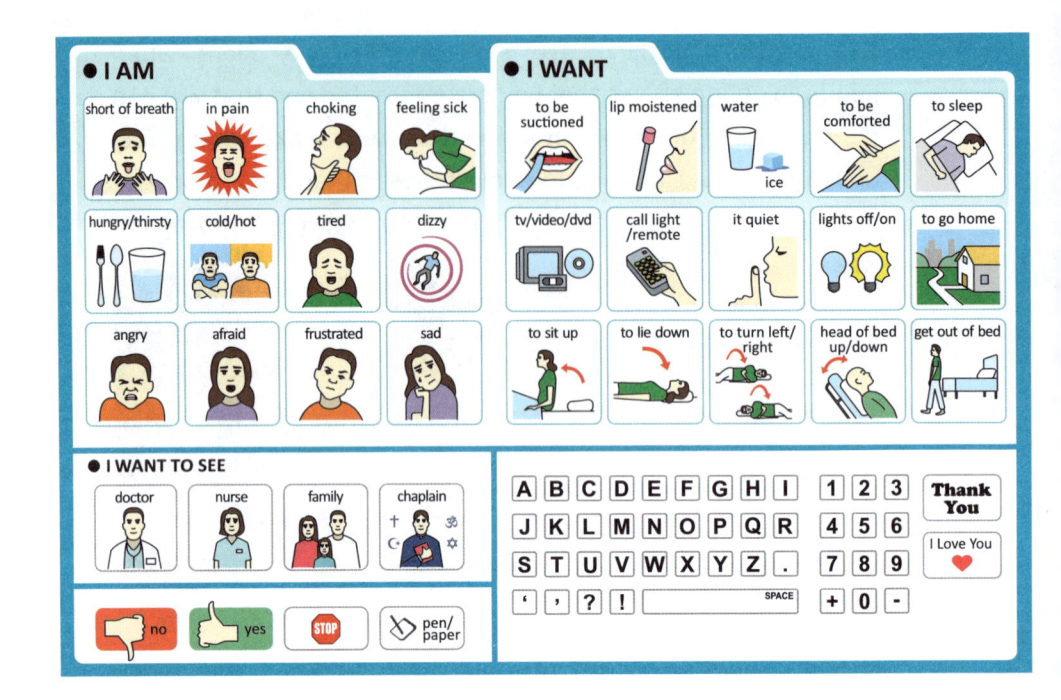

PERSONAL COMMUNICATION TIPS

- Always knock on a client's door and wait for permission before entering.

- When communicating with a client, the first thing you must do is greet them and introduce yourself: 'Hello. My name is ...'

- Always ask for permission and explain, step by step, the care intervention you wish to assist the individual with. In doing this you are offering autonomy and giving control back to the individual.

- Find out how the client would like to be addressed. Don't assume that we can call them by their first name – ask them what they would like to be called. Some people prefer you to call them by their title, e.g. Mrs Murphy. It may seem very formal to us, but we must respect the client's wishes.

- Speak to the client directly. Don't speak over them or leave them out of the conversation. Two carers working together may be tempted to chat away together, about a night out, what they watched on TV last night, etc., but this can make the client feel invisible. Always ask the client questions directly; for example, if they have a relative visiting, don't ask the relative, 'Does he/she take sugar in their tea?', ask the client.

- Don't use your mobile phone at work for non-work matters. Check your workplace policy on mobile phone use and stick to it.

- Avoid using pet names, such as 'love, 'pet', 'my dear'. Some clients don't mind this, but others hate it. If you are looking after adults, speak to them as an adult and don't use baby language. This can belittle the client and is disrespectful.

- Before any cares are given to the client we must have their consent. If they don't give us permission, we mustn't proceed. Where possible, give the client choices.

- Full explanations must be given to the client in a way that they can understand. Always be honest when giving information to clients and you will build a trusting relationship. If a client asks you something and cannot answer, explain that you will ask the nurse in charge or supervisor to come and speak to them.

- We don't just talk to clients about the cares we are giving them, we chat to them. Clients will enjoy chatting. The topic we never tire of talking about in Ireland is the weather! Chatting to the client will help to build a relationship with them. Don't gossip – keep the chat general and don't become over-familiar. We must have a friendly but professional relationship with our clients. Give visitors privacy and never listen in on private phone conversations.

CONFIDENTIALITY

In your work experience placement, you will be asked to sign a confidentiality contract. The client has a right to privacy, so anything concerning their care must be treated as confidential. Client information must only be discussed in appropriate places, with appropriate people, in private. You can discuss cares for the client with your co-workers in the staff-room, but you cannot discuss the client on the bus on your way home from work. Avoid others overhearing when you are passing on information about the client. Reply tactfully to relatives and friends who are looking for information. If there are telephone inquiries, refer them to the supervisor.

BARRIERS TO COMMUNICATION

Sometimes there are barriers to communication. The environment may not be suitable, or there may not be enough privacy, or there may be too many people about. The way you speak to the client can create a barrier, as they may have difficulty understanding you. The client may not hear you if they have impaired hearing or cognitive difficulties. People who are anxious don't always hear what is being said – their anxiety can make it difficult for them to take in the information.

> **Task** Work in groups to think of ways you could overcome these barriers.

COMMUNICATING EFFECTIVELY WITH CLIENTS WITH HEARING PROBLEMS

Many clients with hearing problems find communication in healthcare settings difficult, and this might sometimes affect their care. When conversing with clients with hearing problems, a good communication strategy should include the following:

- Get the client's attention before starting the conversation by calling their name, waving or tapping on their shoulder.
- Introduce the general topic of discussion to the client. It will help the client to know the topic in order to pick up key works. If the topic changes, inform the client.
- Speak at normal speed, but speak distinctly and clearly. Do not shout, exaggerate or over-pronounce words.
- Always look directly at the client when speaking and maintain eye contact for the duration of the conversation.
- Do not place anything in your mouth before or when speaking – be mindful to facilitate, not hinder lipreading.
- Use the words 'I' and 'you' if communicating through an interpreter.
- Do not stand in front of a light source such as a window or bright lighting, as a glare or shadow may impede lipreading.
- If you have problems being understood, repeat your sentences first and then try to rephrase them in a different way.
- Use body language and facial expressions to help your communication.
- Always be courteous and polite to the client during conversation.
- Take turns speaking – never interrupt.
- Provide important information such as dates or numbers in writing.
- Try to read the client's facial expressions and use open-ended questions requiring more than a yes/no answer to ensure that they have understood your message.

COMMUNICATING WITH OTHERS

Family and friends: You will also communicate with the family and friends of the client. Be careful not to reveal confidential information about the client.

Work colleagues: You also will have to communicate with your other work colleagues. Good communication is a very important aspect of teamwork. You are all working together to care for the client, so good communication between work colleagues means that there is good continuity of care. You must treat your work colleagues with respect and act in a professional manner at all times.

Other members of the interdisciplinary team: As we saw in the previous chapter, many people may be involved in caring for the client. Your knowledge and information about the client will help them to deliver good services and care to the client. Good communication is important. Be clear when passing information on. Listen carefully to any instructions and if you are unsure, check what is being said. Be respectful to other members of the interdisciplinary team. They should also treat you with respect.

Case Study

Johnny is a 55-year-old patient in the Accident and Emergency department. He has abdominal (stomach) pain and is waiting for a bed on the surgical ward. He has been in A&E for 26 hours and he has had no sleep or rest. He is a smoker but hasn't had a cigarette since he arrived. He is anxious, and he is beginning to feel angry. He has a drip in his arm and the A&E staff are afraid that, due to his anxiety, he will try to remove it. You are asked to stay with Johnny and keep him calm while he waits for a bed. There should be a bed available in the next two hours, but no one has informed Johnny of this.

+ Explain how you will communicate with Johnny while he is waiting for his bed.

Revision Questions:

1. Define *communication*.
2. What are the different types of non-verbal communication?
3. Why is effective communication in the workplace necessary?
4. Why is confidentiality important?
5. Name two barriers to communication.

Key words/phrases:

active listening

verbal communication

non-verbal communication

confidentiality

DIGNITY AND RESPECT 04

Respecting the dignity of the client and maintaining their privacy is the foundation of care-giving. The clients you are caring for are all unique individuals and deserving of respect. When caring for others, treat them as you would like to be treated or as you would like your loved ones to be treated. We should at all times look after our clients with care and compassion. This is a principle we should never lose sight of.

IN THIS CHAPTER YOU WILL LEARN ABOUT:

- The values needed to care for clients
- Empathy
- How to respectfully care for someone during sensitive procedures while maintaining their privacy
- Promoting independence and empowering the client
- Promoting a positive self-image – feeling good about yourself
- Barriers to respectful care and how to overcome the barriers

VALUES IN ACTION

The HSE programme Values in Action is based on nine behaviours that reflect the values of care, compassion, trust and learning. The nine key behaviours reflect the three dimensions in our working lives: the individual dimension; the work dimension; and the patient dimension.

They are a guide to how to be the best version of ourselves – as individuals, with our colleagues and with our patients. Through Values in Action we can create a better working environment for our colleagues and deliver better experiences to our patients and clients.

The Values in Action behaviours are designed as practical questions that the carer can reflect on as a means of checking that they are working in a caring fashion.

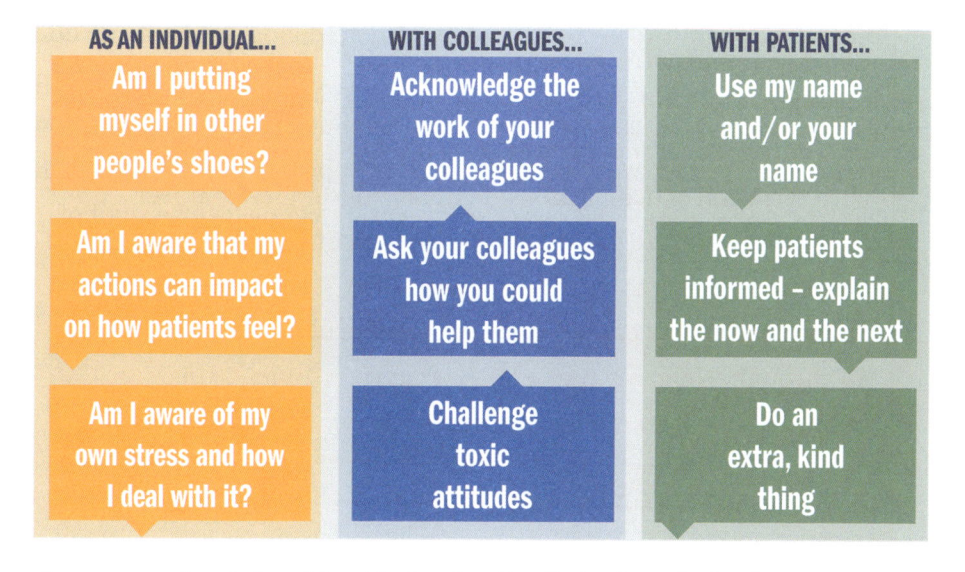

AS AN INDIVIDUAL...	WITH COLLEAGUES...	WITH PATIENTS...
Am I putting myself in other people's shoes?	Acknowledge the work of your colleagues	Use my name and/or your name
Am I aware that my actions can impact on how patients feel?	Ask your colleagues how you could help them	Keep patients informed – explain the now and the next
Am I aware of my own stress and how I deal with it?	Challenge toxic attitudes	Do an extra, kind thing

Source: www.hse.ie/eng/about/valuesinaction/behaviours/behaviours.html

Task Discuss with a classmate what values and characteristics you feel are important when caring for others. How many of these values and characteristics do you possess? Are there any that you feel that you need to work on?

> **Hello, my name is …**
>
> A campaign to encourage healthcare workers to introduce themselves was started by a terminally ill doctor in the UK, who was shocked at how many care-givers failed to introduce themselves. The 'Hello my name is …' campaign was spearheaded by Dr Kate Granger, a young hospital consultant from Yorkshire who worked in elderly care, to improve the patient experience not only in the UK, but across the world. Kate became frustrated with the number of staff who failed to introduce themselves to her when she was in hospital. Dr Granger became a patient herself when she was diagnosed with terminal cancer, and made it her mission in whatever time she had left to get as many members of NHS staff as possible pledging to introduce themselves to their patients. Sadly, Dr Granger passed away on 23 July 2016. Her legacy lives on through 'Hello my name is …', which continues to inspire healthcare staff in the UK and across the world.
>
> This campaign is simple – it reminds staff to go back to basics and introduce themselves to patients properly. Kate talked about this as 'the first rung on the ladder to providing compassionate care' and saw it as the start of making a vital human connection, beginning a therapeutic relationship and building trust between patients and healthcare staff (HSE n.d.).

Maintaining Dignity

It is important that we maintain dignity and respect for clients when attending to personal cares. Examples of sensitive procedures include washing a client or helping them go to the toilet. We all have habits and peculiarities that we may not want to share with others. We all have a private space and feel uncomfortable when others enter this space.

Society also has unwritten rules about touch. When we are caring for someone we have to enter their personal space and we have to touch the client. The first time you have to help a client with a sensitive task, you may feel embarrassed and uncomfortable. You may feel very aware of how embarrassing it might be for the client. After a while, these tasks become part of your daily routine, and you will lose your sense of embarrassment, but be aware that tasks that can become routine to the carer can continue to be distressing and embarrassing for the client. Try to remember what it might be like for them.

When you are assisting with personal cares:

- Knock before entering.
- Introduce yourself – 'Hello, my name is …'
- Ask the client what they wish to be called – don't assume.
- Always get consent for any procedures.
- Give full explanations and give choices. Involve the client in decision-making.
- Always ensure privacy. Close curtains and doors.
- Keep as much of the body covered as possible during procedures.
- Never express disgust. Be aware of your facial expressions.
- Speak in a quiet voice when asking sensitive questions.
- Be sensitive to different cultural practices.
- Always encourage the independence of the individual – positive reinforcement.

EMPATHY

Empathy is the ability to be sensitive to others' needs and communicate an understanding of their feelings – putting yourself in another's shoes. It involves listening, good communication (and appropriate use of silence), reflection, touch, respect and compassion. It can be conveyed both verbally and non-verbally. Empathy is different from sympathy, which is feeling compassion, sorrow or pity for the hardships of another person.

SYMPATHY

I'm sorry — that sucks.

EMPATHY

Being empathetic towards a client encourages the client to share the burden of their fears and anxieties. Listening intently to a client's concerns or fears creates a trust between carer and client, which can lead to a bond being created. Acknowledging and affirming a client's suffering can lead to a sense of empowerment for the client, resulting in renewed or greater strength and determination to face their future (Sealy 2011).

When engaging with a client and discussing their concerns, be aware of the following.

+ **Eye contact** is extremely important.
+ **Use facial expressions** and nod your head, be physically close but respect their space, make positive hand gestures, have

an open posture, and lean forward slightly to indicate your attentiveness and willingness to engage.

- **Do not write notes** or read a chart during a difficult conversation or when dealing with a client's emotions.

- **You can show distress** if you feel it, but be genuine and ensure that your emotions are caused by your client's circumstance and not your own personal issues.

- **Do not** let your emotions affect your decision-making.

The NURSE mnemonic is a useful aid to help you respond appropriately to clients' emotions.

- **N – Name it.** 'It sounds like you've been worried about what's going on ...'

- **U – Understand** the core message. 'If I understand you correctly, you're worried about what to say to your family and how they will react?'

- **R – Respect/Reassurance** at the right time: 'I'm really impressed that you've continued to be independent.'

- **S – Support.** 'Would you like me to talk to your family about ...?'

- **E – Explore.** 'I notice that you're upset – can you tell me what you're thinking?' (Back *et al.* 2009).

PROMOTING INDEPENDENCE

Gently encourage the client to do as much as they can for themselves. For example, when helping them with their hygiene, let them wash their own face and hands. The client will feel better about themselves if they are allowed to be independent. It will make them feel in control. Encourage the client without being bossy or domineering. Allow them time and don't rush them.

> **Task** Discuss in groups the different ways in which you can promote independence. Think of practical examples.

PROMOTING A POSITIVE SELF-IMAGE

Feeling valued and respected makes us feel good about ourselves. Clients who need assistance with day-to-day activities may feel as though they are a burden or a nuisance. We can avoid this by treating them with respect and communicating clearly with them.

Introduce yourself. Give them explanations and choices and don't take away their independence or autonomy. Be friendly and interested in them. Smile. Give them compliments. Ensure that they are clean and neatly dressed. How we dress and look can have a positive effect on our self-image. Allow them to dress in their choice of clothes, and respect individual choices. If they want to wear make-up or jewellery, assist them if necessary. Having their hair done will make them feel good. The care setting may have pampering sessions, with manicures and pedicures.

You need to attend to all the needs of the client – physical, emotional, social, intellectual and spiritual. Listen to the client if they are upset or anxious. Ensure that they can socialise and mix with others and take part in interests and hobbies, which will help with their self-worth. For some clients, religious beliefs underpin who they feel they are. We must ensure that all the needs are seen to and that the whole person is cared for as an individual.

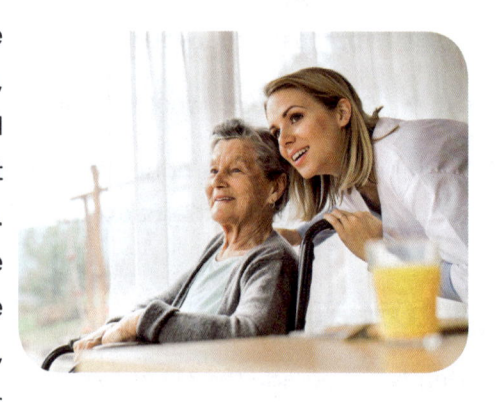

THE CLIENT'S PERSONAL SPACE

The client's personal space should reflect them as an individual. Allow them to display photos and pictures, religious objects, memorabilia, curios or gifts representing their life, family and wider community.

> **Task** Can you suggest other ways of promoting a positive self-image?

BARRIERS

There are barriers and difficulties in providing respectful individualised care, the biggest ones being lack of time and low staffing levels. In some settings clients do not have their own private space and they may have to share their room. The client may feel anxious, which can prevent a person hearing what is being communicated. These barriers can be challenging, and plans should be put in place to overcome them.

Caring for the client in a respectful manner should be the guiding principle when working as a carer. Flexibility is very important when caring for clients. Too much routine – e.g. getting clients up early in the morning and back to bed early in the day, all washes taking place in the morning, toileting done at certain times, meal times early in the day etc. – can be seen as elements of institutionalised care. Some clients may not want to shower in the morning, so be flexible.

Even when you are busy, try to make friendly contact with your client. Chatting to them isn't wasting time; it's just as valuable as attending to their hygiene needs. Make the most of the time you spend helping with a client's needs by chatting to them and showing that you are interested in them as an individual.

Exercise:

Roisin is 19 years old and lives with cerebral palsy. She is wheelchair bound and needs assistance with some of her physical cares, but manages to live a full and active life. She has participated in mainstream secondary school with the help of a special needs assistant. She is hoping to go to the graduation dinner and dance but is feeling anxious about attending.

+ Explain how her carer will deal with this.

Revision Questions:

1. What are the nine behaviours in the HSE programme Values in Action?
2. What is empathy?
3. List three ways in which you would promote a client's positive self-image.
4. What are the barriers to showing a client respect and dignity?

Key words/phrases:

compassion

positive self-image

empathy

sympathy

personal space

dignity

respect

HYGIENE

05

Carers often have to help people to do the day-to-day things we all do every day. Some clients are highly dependent on others to see to these activities. They may need help to wash themselves, to attend to their grooming needs, to dress, to go to the toilet, to mobilise, to eat and drink, and they may even need assistance with their social needs. In this chapter, we will look at how we can help with an individual's hygiene needs – how to assist them with washing.

IN THIS CHAPTER YOU WILL LEARN ABOUT:

- The importance of personal hygiene and dress code
- The appropriate use of personal protective equipment (PPE)
- The importance of hand hygiene
- The importance of communication in hygiene assistance
- Planning and preparation – prepare the client, yourself and the environment
- Adapting the level of help to the individual
- After-care procedures
- The importance of the individual when assisting with hygiene
- How to maintain the respect and dignity of the person
- Being aware of cultural considerations
- How to report and record cares given

THE CLIENT'S HYGIENE NEEDS

Some clients you will be caring for will need help getting washed. Not everyone will need the same level of assistance. The help that you give depends on the individual needs of the person you are caring for. When you are caring for someone you need to follow certain steps.

1. Plan and prepare before you start.

2. Perform the care skill safely, and maintain good hygiene standards.

3. Ensure that you communicate effectively throughout, maintaining the dignity and respect of the person being cared for.

4. Afterwards, tidy up and safely clean and store any equipment used.

5. Report and document the cares given.

Consultation and Assessment

First determine how much assistance is needed by checking the care plans. A **care plan** is a written document that details the assistance the individual person may need and how this care should be given. This care plan may be kept in a filing cabinet in the office or in some cases on a computer.

You may have been given a spoken handover at the start of the work shift. Be aware that any notes you make during handover may contain confidential information. Make yourself familiar with your workplace's policies on **data protection**. The confidentiality of the person must always be maintained.

Consult with the person you are caring for and ask what help they need and how you can help them. Planning allows you to adapt the level of care to the individual needs of the person.

THE CARER AND HYGIENE STANDARDS

The carer must follow good hygiene standards to reduce the risk of spreading infections. The carer must follow dress code, hand hygiene guidelines and must use PPE appropriately.

HYGIENE PLANNING AND PREPARATION

Preparing Yourself

Dress Code

You should always be dressed appropriately and in accordance with the policies of your workplace. The guiding principles are that you maintain safety and good hygiene.

- Footwear should be flat, non-slip and comfortable as you will be on your feet most of the working day.
- Wear soft-soled shoes as they reduce noise, which can disturb patients' rest.
- Avoid open-toed sandals as they will not protect your feet against spills.
- Hair must be kept up off the face.
- Nails should be clean and short as sharp nails may scrape the person being cared for. Don't wear false nails or nail varnish.
- Keep any cuts or abrasions covered.

- Changing into a clean uniform at the start of each shift prevents any risk of cross-contamination and bringing in germs from home.

- Wear a short-sleeved top/shirt. Cuffs become heavily contaminated and are more likely to come into contact with the client.

- Change immediately if clothes become heavily soiled or contaminated.

- Wash uniforms at the hottest programme suitable for the fabric. Washing for 10 minutes at 60°C removes most organisms.

- Do not wear jewellery – it can harbour germs that may spread infections. Sharp jewellery can potentially scratch or scrape the person you are caring for, while long dangly earrings or necklaces could be grabbed, causing strangulation or injury. Most workplaces will allow only stud earrings and a wedding band.

- **Not recommended:** Wearing neckties – they are worn daily but rarely laundered. They have been shown to be colonised by harmful germs (HSE Standard Precautions).

Personal Protective Equipment (PPE)

Personal protective equipment (PPE) is the equipment we use to protect ourselves from potential hazards in the workplace. The PPE that carers use most often is gloves and aprons. They are worn for most of the care tasks carried out with the client.

- Gloves reduce the risk of exposure of staff to body fluids and protect clients from organisms that may be on healthcare workers' hands. However, they won't protect clients if they are not changed between clients, so remember to change gloves and aprons and to wash hands between clients.

- Staff with a latex allergy must be provided with alternatives, e.g. nitrile or vinyl gloves.

CHAPTER 05: HYGIENE 49

+ Always wash your hands before and after putting on gloves. Wearing gloves is never a substitute for good hand hygiene!

+ Perform a risk assessment – if you don't need gloves, don't wear them.

+ Gloves should be put on by holding the wrist end of the glove open with one hand to allow the other hand to enter easily. Gloves are single-use items. They are put on immediately before an episode of patient contact or treatment and removed as soon as the activity is completed. The same PPE should never be worn for a different patient, client, procedure or area.

+ Disposable plastic aprons prevent blood/body fluid splashes getting on to clothes or skin.

+ Discard gloves and aprons safely and attend to hand hygiene.

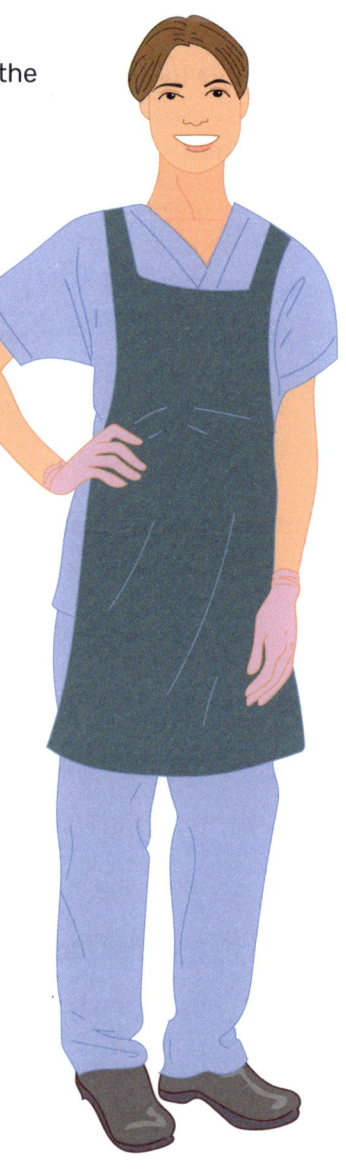

Hand Hygiene

Hand washing is one of the most important steps in preventing the spread of infection. Carers have an important role in keeping clients safe as they are the ones that have the most interaction with clients.

Hands must be washed:

- **When –**
    - visibly dirty or soiled
    - between different types of cleaning procedures.

- **Before –**
    - starting work, going for a break, and leaving for home
    - any cleaning task
    - preparing or handling food and drinks and/or when handling any other related catering equipment
    - entering and leaving an isolation area.

- **After –**
    - handling any item that is soiled
    - handling linen, bedding and waste
    - removing any protective clothing including gloves
    - any cleaning task
    - using the toilet
    - blowing the nose (RCPI/HSE 2012).

The WHO identifies five moments when it is essential to attend to hand hygiene.

CHAPTER 05: HYGIENE

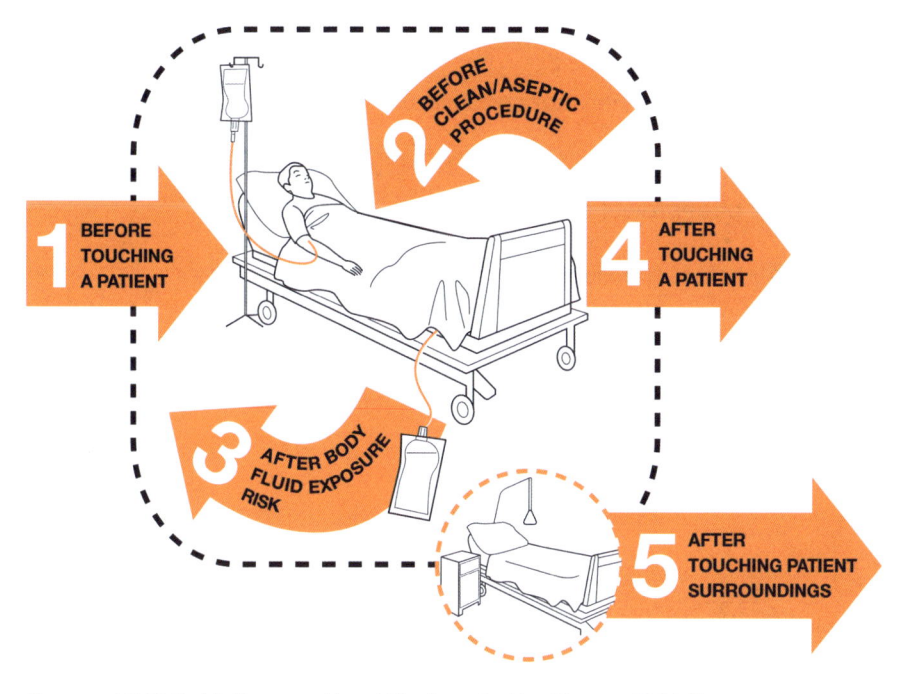

Source: WHO Guidelines on Hand Hygiene in Healthcare (2009)

An alcohol hand rub can be used for hand hygiene, *except* in the following situations, when hands must be washed with soap and water:

+ when hands are visibly soiled

+ when caring for patients known or suspected to have *Clostridium difficile* infection.

Hand-washing Procedure: Soap and Water

+ Wet hands under running water.

+ Avoid using over-hot water.

+ Apply enough liquid or foam soap to cover all surfaces of the hands and wrists.

+ The soap solution must come into contact with all surfaces of the hands and wrists.

COMPLETE CARE SKILLS

- Rub hands together vigorously for at least 15 seconds.
- Rinse hands thoroughly.
- Do not use clean hands to turn off tap. If taps are not hands-free, use paper towel to turn off tap.
- Dry hands thoroughly with disposable paper towels.
- Discard towel in hands-free non-risk waste bin.

Hand Hygiene Technique with Soap and Water

Duration of the entire procedure: 40-60 seconds

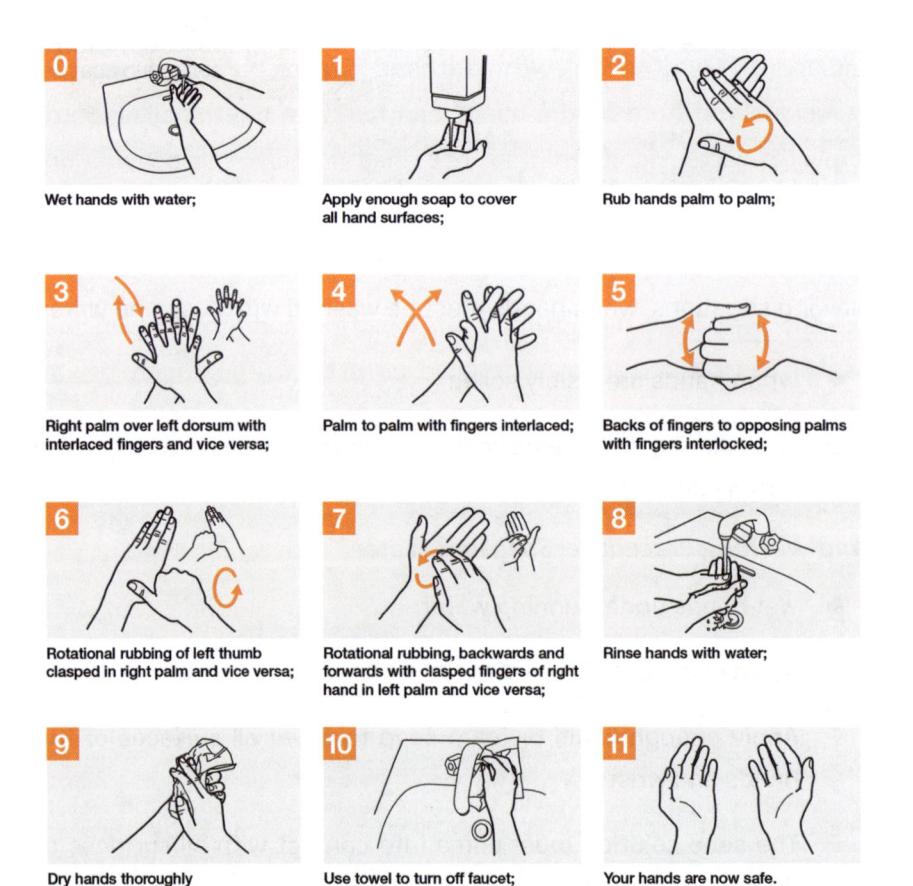

0 Wet hands with water;

1 Apply enough soap to cover all hand surfaces;

2 Rub hands palm to palm;

3 Right palm over left dorsum with interlaced fingers and vice versa;

4 Palm to palm with fingers interlaced;

5 Backs of fingers to opposing palms with fingers interlocked;

6 Rotational rubbing of left thumb clasped in right palm and vice versa;

7 Rotational rubbing, backwards and forwards with clasped fingers of right hand in left palm and vice versa;

8 Rinse hands with water;

9 Dry hands thoroughly with a single use towel;

10 Use towel to turn off faucet;

11 Your hands are now safe.

Source: WHO Guidelines on Hand Hygiene in Healthcare (2009)

Notes:

1. Nailbrushes should *not* be used to clean the hands, as scrubbing can break the skin, leading to an increased risk of harbouring micro-organisms or dispersing skin scales. Where nailbrushes are used for surgical scrub they should be fit for purpose and single use.

2. Bar soap should *not* be used by staff for hand hygiene in a clinical or care setting. It is acceptable for a client's own use but not for sharing between clients.

Hand Drying

Hand drying plays a critical role in the hand hygiene procedure because any residual moisture on the hands can facilitate the transmission of micro-organisms. Hands that are not dried properly can become dry and cracked, leading to an increased risk of harbouring micro-organisms.

Once the taps have been turned off using a 'hands-free' technique, clean disposable paper towels should be used to thoroughly dry all areas of the hands. This should be done by drying each part of the hand following the steps recommended for hand washing. Soft, user-friendly, disposable paper towels are best.

Alcohol-based Hand Rub Procedure

- Do not use alcohol hand rub on visibly soiled hands.
- The amount needed to cover the hands adequately should be given in the manufacturer's instructions. It is normally around 3 ml.
- Follow the same steps as for hand washing with soap and water.
- The hand rub solution must come into contact with all surfaces of the hands and wrists.

✚ Rub hands together vigorously for at least 15 seconds until the solution has evaporated and hands are dry. Some manufacturers recommend rubbing for 30 seconds – check the label.

Hand Hygiene Technique with Alcohol-Based Formulation

🕐 **Duration of the entire procedure:** 20-30 seconds

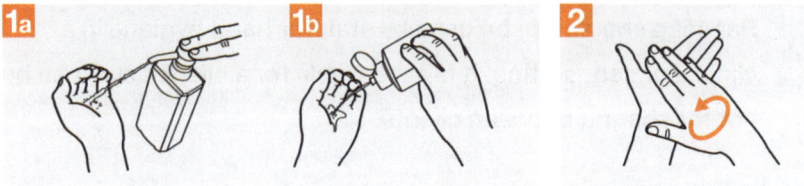

1a / 1b Apply a palmful of the product in a cupped hand, covering all surfaces;

2 Rub hands palm to palm;

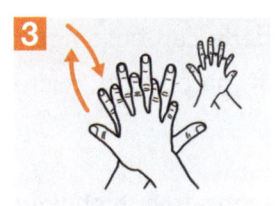

3 Right palm over left dorsum with interlaced fingers and vice versa;

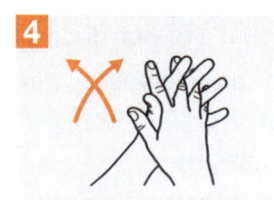

4 Palm to palm with fingers interlaced;

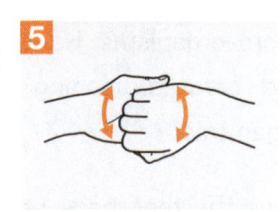

5 Backs of fingers to opposing palms with fingers interlocked;

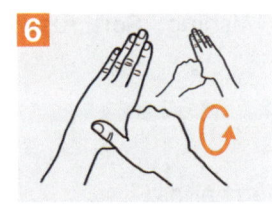

6 Rotational rubbing of left thumb clasped in right palm and vice versa;

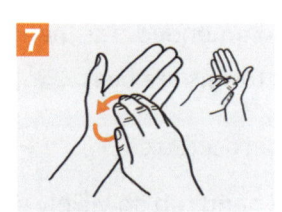

7 Rotational rubbing, backwards and forwards with clasped fingers of right hand in left palm and vice versa;

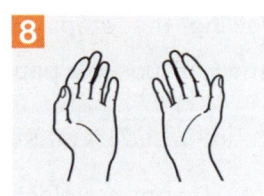

8 Once dry, your hands are safe.

Source: WHO Guidelines on Hand Hygiene in Healthcare (2009)

Hand Care

It is important to protect the skin from drying and cracking. Cracked skin can harbour micro-organisms and broken skin can become contaminated, particularly when exposed to blood and body fluids.

CHAPTER 05: HYGIENE

Handcreams can be applied to the skin, but only individual tubes of handcream for single-person use or handcream from wall-mounted dispensers should be used. Communal tubs must be avoided as they can collect bacteria over time, and lead to contamination of hands.

Remember!

- Poor hand hygiene is one of the leading causes of the spread of infection in the workplace.

- The correct hand hygiene procedure should be followed and at the appropriate times.

- Always attend to hand hygiene between clients.

- Liquid soap and water or alcohol hand rub may be used for hand hygiene. In some cases, alcohol hand rub is not effective (see section on Hygiene).

- If using soap and water, the soap must be from a dispenser.

- The sink tap(s) should not be touched following hand washing. The taps may be operated by a sensor, or with a long handle that can be turned with your elbows. If neither is available, use disposable towels to turn off the taps.

- Dry hands thoroughly using disposable towels and put the used towels in a touch-free bin, in other words a pedal bin, to avoid touching the bin lid with your hands.

- Frequent hand washing can lead to sore and cracked skin as the detergents in the soaps also strip away the skin's natural oils. Using handcream can help prevent this. Your workplace should have handcream available near the hand washing facilities.

Task Practise hand hygiene in the classroom.

Preparing the Client

Always knock before entering the room. When you go in, say hello, smile, and introduce yourself.

Discuss

Reflection: How would you feel if somebody entered your bedroom, didn't speak to you or tell you who they were and started removing your clothes and washing you? You would feel violated. So always remember to treat people as you would like to be treated and cared for.

Task

Roleplay. Practise your introduction and greeting with the person beside you.

You must always keep the client informed about their care. This means explaining all procedures to them. It is important to talk to the person and tell them what you are doing even if they don't seem to understand. No cares can be given without consent. If the person refuses care, you cannot give that care.

Discuss

What do you think you should do if you feel the person needs to have a shower, but that person is angrily refusing a wash?

Preparing the Environment

Make the room safe for the task and make it comfortable for the client and for yourself. The privacy of the person being assisted with their hygiene needs must be maintained. If there are visitors present, politely ask them to leave. Pull curtains and close doors. In hospital settings and some nursing home settings the rooms are shared, and sometimes all that separates the clients is a curtain. Don't forget that curtains are not sound-proof! Be sensitive when communicating with the client and be aware that others in the room may hear everything.

CHAPTER 05: HYGIENE

Close windows to avoid a draught.

Move furniture carefully if necessary. Make room for yourself; don't do the task if you would have to twist and move around obstacles. Nursing homes and hospitals will have height-adjustable beds, so raise the bed to hip level so that you don't need to bend over the person. If there are bed rails, lower them or move the bed if necessary. Remember, repetitive movements can be harmful to your back.

> **Bed Rails: Safety Note**
>
> Bed rails should only be used if they are suitable for the individual client. If bed rails are used inappropriately they can be a danger to the client – they may be confused, try to get out of bed, climb over the rails and fall. If the client is restless they may trap their legs and get cuts and lacerations; in the worst-case scenario the bed rails can cause strangulation. Bed rail can be used for some clients, but only after a risk assessment is completed.

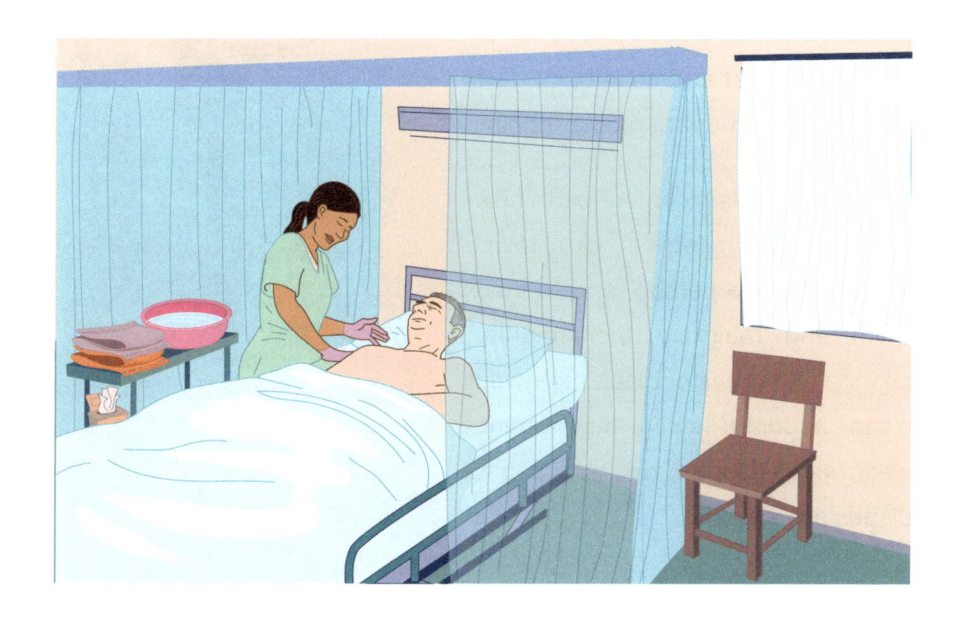

EQUIPMENT

A number of pieces of equipment are used to assist with hygiene.

Washing Aids

Several aids are available to help a client attend to their hygiene and grooming needs.

- Shower chairs, to allow the client to sit while showering.
- A railing in the shower will help the client to keep their balance.
- Non-slip flooring is very important.
- Long-handled sponges allow the client to wash independently and clean hard-to-reach areas.
- Special tap handles make it easier to turn taps on and off.

If the person has been assessed as needing assistance with movement, a hoist may be necessary. Ensure that you have been properly trained in the use of the hoist and have been given manual and patient handling training.

Other essentials include a wash bowl, warm water, toiletries, two towels (one to dry the person, one to cover them and maintain their dignity), change of clothes or clean nightwear, clean bedding, clean incontinence wear, wipes, laundry bag, and bag for disposing of waste.

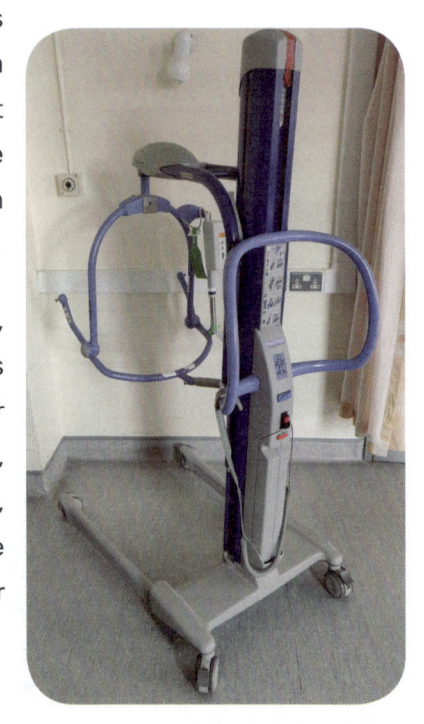

CHAPTER 05: HYGIENE

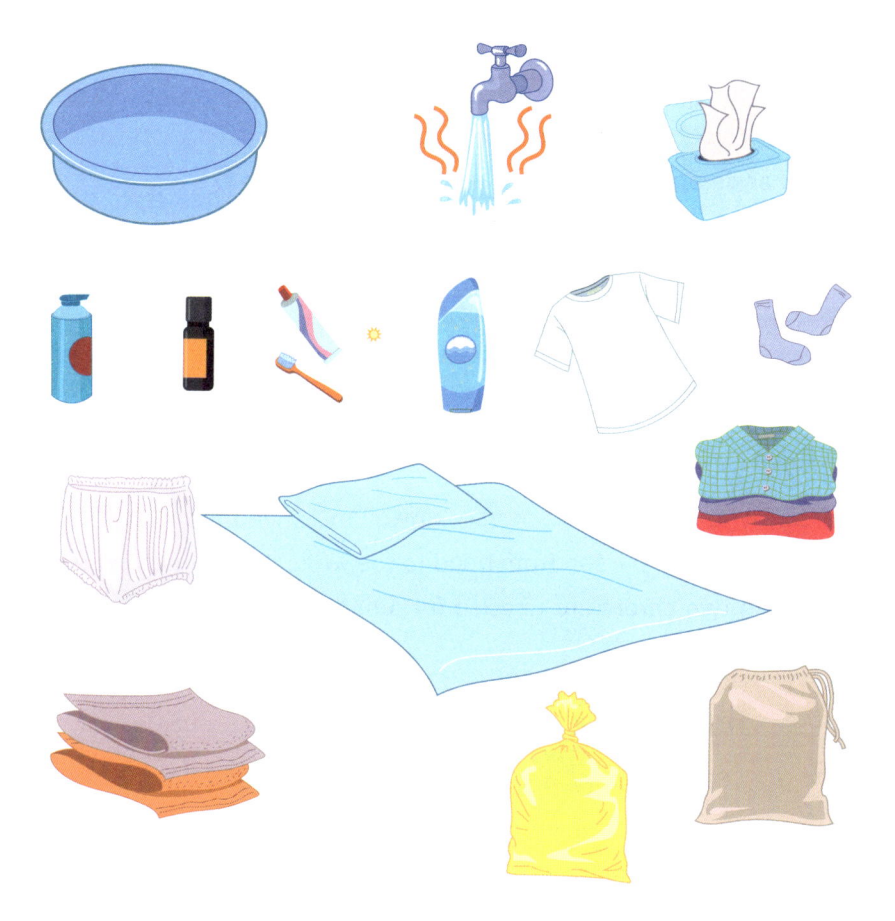

The equipment you need will depend on your workplace and on the type of hygiene assistance given. If you are working in the person's own home, you will need to use what is available in the home.

Finally, determine how many carers are needed. Heavily dependent clients will need two or even three carers to assist with their hygiene needs.

TYPES OF ASSISTANCE

Not everyone you are caring for will need the same level of assistance. Even two people with a similar condition may need different levels of assistance. Treat every person as an individual. You are not performing a list of tasks that are the same for everyone. Adapt the level of assistance given to the person needing the assistance.

Types of assistance:

- bed bath
- assisted wash
- shower or bath.

Bed Bath

A person who is bedbound or very unwell may need a bed bath. This involves washing a person from head to toe while they remain in bed. In most cases two carers are needed for a bed bath – one carer washes and the other dries.

Tips for Giving a Bed Bath

- Wear gloves if there is any chance that you might come in contact with blood or other body fluids.
- Keep your client covered during the bed bath except for the area you are cleaning. This helps keep them from getting chilled and preserves their dignity.
- Wash the cleaner areas of the body first and the dirtier areas last to help reduce the spread of germs.
- Place a towel under the part of the body being washed. This will absorb any excess bath water and keep the bed sheets dry.
- Wash and dry thoroughly between folds of the skin.
- Keep the washcloth wet, but not so wet that it drips.
- Only use a mild soap and always remove all soap residue.
- Dry the skin after it has been rinsed.

- Replace the water if it cools during the bath.
- Apply lotion to the skin after bathing to prevent the skin drying.

There are different ways of doing a bed bath, so follow your workplace guidelines.

Give clear explanations to your client and always get consent. The client needing the bed bath may be able to do things for him/herself. Encourage them to do what they can, e.g. wash their hands and face. This will encourage independence and boost their self-esteem, even if it does take more time. Give the client some personal choices, such as choosing a nightdress or pyjamas.

> **Eyes**
>
> Some people need to have their eyes carefully cleaned during the wash. Use cotton wool swabs and sterile water to carefully clean eyes, wiping from the inside of the eye to the outside. Discard used swabs and use a clean swab for each wipe.

Bed Bath: Suggested Routine

- Fill a basin with warm water and place on a table next to the bed.
- Beginning with the head, wipe the patient's eyes, from the nose towards the ear, with cotton wool (gauze) swabs and sterile water, wiping from the inside of the eye to the outside. Discard used swabs.
- Lather the cloth with mild soap and wash the face and neck.
- Rinse the washcloth and remove soapy residue from the skin; dry well.

COMPLETE CARE SKILLS

- Bathe each arm separately, rinse off soapy residue and dry.

- For a thorough hand washing, place the hand in the basin of water while washing it.

- Wash the chest, abdomen, each leg, and then feet, rinse off soapy residue and dry. Clean the genital area by folding the washcloth into a mitt and gently wiping area with a small amount of soapy water. Rinse away soapy residue and dry area.

- Help your client onto his or her side.

- Wash and dry their back.

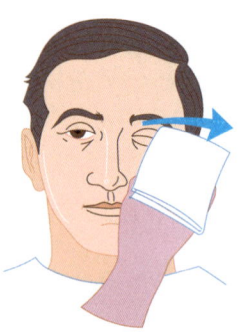

Wash the eyes first. From the inside corner to the outside, using a different area of the cloth for each eye.

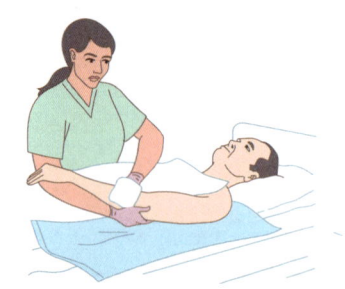

After washing the face, neck, and ears, remove the gown and wash the arms one at a time.

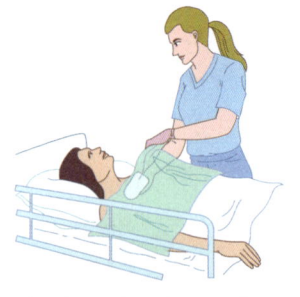

Place the towel over the patient's chest. Lift the corner as you wash the chest. Repeat for the abdomen.

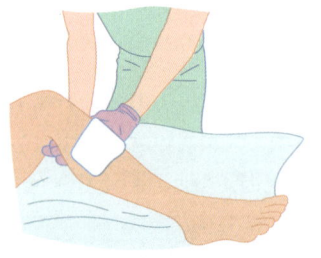

Wash and dry one leg at a time.
Change the water at this time if you have not already needed to do so.

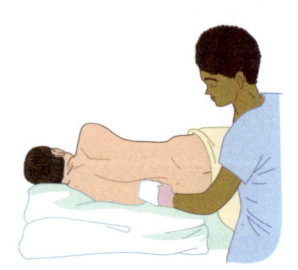

Wash the back and the buttocks.

A bed bath is a good opportunity to check the client's skin for dryness or any sores. Specific areas to pay attention to are: under the breasts – which can become red and sore; buttocks and sacral area; heels; any bony prominences (to check for pressure sores). Pay attention to dry or cracked skin and moisturise if necessary. If the client is wearing anti-embolic stockings, which some clients with reduced mobility wear to help prevent clots forming in the legs, remove during the bed bath and place clean ones on the client after the bed bath.

If you need to use the hoist, make sure that you have been trained in how to use it.

Bed linen can be changed during the bed bath, by rolling the client or by raising the client in the hoist.

Assisted Wash

Some clients only need a small amount of assistance with their hygiene needs. They may need a bowl of water by their bedside and then they can manage to attend to their own needs, or they may need to be helped to the bathroom and they can wash at the sink. Offer any assistance needed with hard-to-reach areas, e.g. back or feet. If this is all the assistance they need, ensure that they have all the equipment necessary and that they have access to a nurse-call button.

Shower or Bath

If there is an option of a shower or a bath, give the client the choice. You must always have the client's consent before you shower or bath them. Remember, if your client is elderly, they may not shower and bath as often as younger generations. Most of us have a shower every day, but this may not be the case for your client. We shouldn't force our ideas of hygiene on another person. Showering can be stressful for some older people, as it makes them feel cold and vulnerable. Some nursing homes keep records of showering and bathing to ensure that clients are regularly showered. However, it is important that the needs and wishes of the clients aren't forgotten – showers or baths should only be given with client agreement and not because the records say they must have a shower on a Tuesday.

The level of assistance needed with showering and bathing depends on the person. Some clients need full assistance in the shower or bath; others will only need to be assisted to the shower. Make sure that they have access to a nurse-call button.

Showering/Bathing Tips

- The bath or shower is likely to be designed to make it easier for the client to enter. Some baths have a watertight door that can be opened, which means that the client doesn't have to climb into the bath. There may also be a special bath hoist to help the client into the bath.

- Many showers you will find in the workplace are designed for wheelchair use and are large enough for the client and the carer. You will probably get wet when assisting with a shower, so use any protective equipment available, such as aprons, overshoes, gloves.

- Bring everything to the shower before you start. Never leave a vulnerable client on their own in the shower or bath.

- Mind yourself – take care not to slip or to injure your back.

- The shower/bath should have grab rails to help the client with standing. Shower or bath chairs can be used. The flooring should be non-slip.

- Showering and bathing is a good time to observe the client's skin and observe their movement. It is also a good time to chat to them and help put them at ease.

CHAPTER 05: HYGIENE

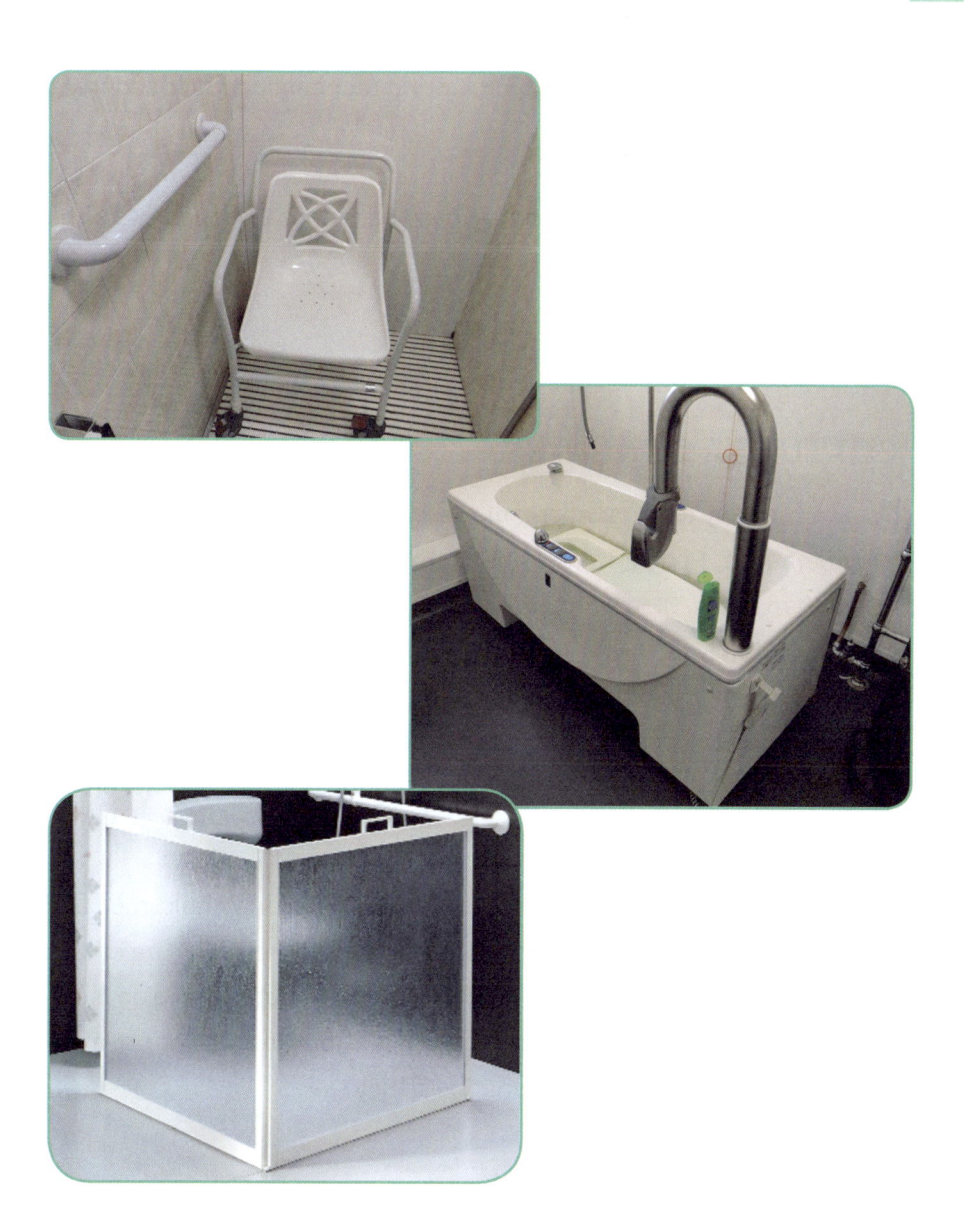

After attending to hygiene needs:

- Clean, tidy and store all equipment.
- Dispose of all waste safely and appropriately.
- Place soiled laundry in the laundry bag.

- Remove gloves and apron following recommended procedure.
- Attend to hand hygiene.
- Record cares given and report any changes or concerns to the nurse in charge.
- Complete any documentation.

CULTURAL CONSIDERATIONS

Be aware of any cultural needs of the client when assisting with their hygiene needs. People from some cultures prefer to wash in showers rather than baths. Older women from some cultures may be traditionally modest and may not want to be washed by a male carer. When caring for someone from a different culture or tradition you should familiarise yourself with the basis of their beliefs and traditions. Refer to the HSE's comprehensive *Health Services: Intercultural Guide*, available on its website (www.hse.ie) (HSE 2009).

Never make assumptions about another person's cultures and traditions. Many of us interpret and adapt our religious beliefs in different ways. We may be very strict on some aspects of religion, such as attending a religious service every week, but less strict on other aspects. Always ask the client what help they want.

AFTERCARE

Make sure the client is dry and warm. Help them return to their bed or their chair. Safely dispose of any waste, categorise dirty linen and place in appropriate linen bags for laundering. Clean any equipment used and store it safely. Tidy up the area. Ensure that the client is happy with the assistance given and that they are content and relaxed.

CHAPTER 05: HYGIENE

Safely remove any PPE and attend to your own hand hygiene.

> **Exercise:**
>
> You are asked to assist an 86-year-old man, John, with his hygiene needs. John has limited mobility due to Parkinson's disease. When you go to John you see that he has spilled his breakfast over his clothes.
>
> + How will you decide what level of assistance John needs?
> + Explain step by step how you will assist John to have a wash.

Remember the Steps

1. **Plan and prepare:** yourself, the client, the environment. Gather your equipment.

2. **Implementing:** remember safety and hygiene.

3. **Person-centred care:** remember that your client is at the centre of your care – give explanations, promote dignity and respect, treat them as an individual, encourage independence, be aware of any cultural considerations.

4. **Aftercare:** safely dispose of waste, store equipment safely, tidy up.

5. **Reporting:** document what cares have been given, report to your supervisor.

Revision Questions:

1. Why is personal hygiene important in the care setting?
2. Why is dress code important?
3. List the different types of hygiene assistance a client might require.
4. Why is hand hygiene important?
5. Why do we record and report information relating to the client?

Key words/phrases:

care plans

data protection

dress code

hand hygiene

hand washing

hand drying

alcohol-based hand rub

personal protective equipment (PPE)

GROOMING, DRESSING AND SENSORY NEEDS 06

Once the client has had their wash or shower, they will want to attend to other needs, such as brushing their hair, shaving, cleaning their teeth, seeing to their hands and feet, and perhaps putting on make-up. They will also want to dress. This will help the person you are caring for to feel good about themselves. Things like the clothes we wear, our hair and make-up, having a shave or trimming a beard are a part of our sense of who we are – our self-identity. They help us to feel like a unique individual. In addition to general grooming and dressing, a client must use any sensory equipment prescribed for them to allow them to fully engage with and interact with their friends, family, carers and wider community.

IN THIS CHAPTER YOU WILL LEARN ABOUT:

- Different types of sensory equipment
- How to use sensory equipment
- How to look after a client's hair
- How to attend to mouth and dental care
- Assisting with shaving
- Assisting with make-up
- How to attend to nail care
- How to assist a client with dressing, with consideration of promoting independence
- The use of care aids to assist the client with grooming and dressing
- Cultural considerations

USE OF SENSORY EQUIPMENT

Sensory equipment is used to help the client see and hear. While attending to the client's grooming and dressing needs and preferences, it is important to ensure that any sensory equipment that the client uses and needs is accessible and in working condition.

Sight

You may have to care for a person with vision impairment; either partial or complete vision loss. If the client wears glasses, make sure they have access to their glasses and that they are clean. A person with vision impairment may be able to read Braille, which is a system of touch reading and writing for blind people in which raised dots represent the letters of the alphabet. Braille readers can also use Braille apps. Occupational therapists will be able to advise clients with vision impairment about the availability of apps.

Other aids that can help a person with vision impairment include magnifying glasses, large print books, audio books, computers that speak (voice activation) and tailored computer programs.

Hearing

Some of your clients may be deaf or hard of hearing. They may have partial or total loss of hearing in both ears or just one ear. There is a wide range of aids that can be used to assist the client.

Hearing aids are small devices, worn in the ear, that amplify sounds for the wearer. A common type of hearing aid is one that loops over the ear with the ear mould going into the ear. You may have to help the client put in their hearing aid, so ensure that the ear mould is correctly inserted into the ear and the hearing aid (which is attached to the ear mould) is placed over the ear. Make sure that the hearing aid is turned on and in good working condition.

CHAPTER 06: GROOMING, DRESSING AND SENSORY NEEDS

Everyday items that can be purchased with modification to suit those with sight and hearing impairments include: alarm clocks that flash and vibrate; talking clocks with calendars; and talking watches – all of which help orient the client to time and place. Doorbells and telephones that flash will alert the person. For children, there are books and DVDs that are illustrated with sign language and use of these books will help a deaf child feel included.

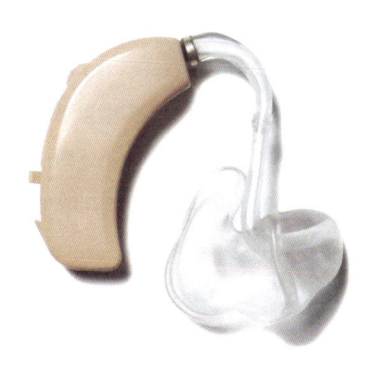

GROOMING

Planning and Preparing Yourself, Your Client and the Environment

- Before attending to grooming, prepare yourself by attending to hand hygiene, and wear the appropriate PPE.

- Prepare the person being cared for by first introducing yourself with 'Hello, my name is …', then get their consent and give explanations throughout the procedures. Ensure that the client is in a good position for grooming.

- Grooming should be done in privacy or in the client's own bedroom or bathroom.

- Prepare the environment by making it safe and secure for you and the client. Gather any equipment needed.

Hair

Comb or brush the hair following the wash. The client may be able to attend to their own needs if they have access to combs, brushes and mirrors. Long-handled combs can be used by the client – this will encourage independence.

The client's hair can be easily washed when they are in the shower, but if they are bedbound it is still possible to wash the hair. Dry shampoos may also be an option; these contain a powder-like substance that soaks up the grease and dirt in the hair, which is then combed out. How often the hair is washed depends on the individual and on the hair.

> **Task** Research ways in which a bedbound person's hair can be washed.

Some care settings have hairdressing facilities. Don't forget that having your hair done can have a positive effect on your feeling of self-esteem and confidence. Going to the hairdressers may have been a regular treat for your client, and many older women will wish to continue with this routine.

Teeth

We need to brush our teeth twice a day. Ensure that your client has access to toothbrushing facilities. If they can brush their own teeth, then encourage independence. Some clients will need help, so use a soft or medium toothbrush with a small head and toothpaste to carefully brush the client's teeth. Brush all surfaces of the teeth.

There are special toothbrushes available to help brush the teeth of clients who have limited ability to co-operate. A three-headed toothbrush is designed to brush the three surfaces of the teeth at the same time. Some people may use an electric toothbrush. Non-foaming toothpaste can be used on clients unable to spit out toothpaste.

CHAPTER 06: GROOMING, DRESSING AND SENSORY NEEDS

A toothbrush needs to be replaced every three months. Check to see if the bristles are becoming worn. Store the toothbrush safely and label it with the client's name. It is important that toothbrushes are not shared between clients.

Allow them to rinse their mouth afterwards and have a bowl for them to spit into.

Some clients may wear **dentures**, which are removable false teeth, and which also need to be washed daily. If the client is unable to wash their own dentures, you will have to clean them. Clean with a toothbrush and denture cream. Regular toothpaste is too abrasive for dentures and can damage them. Some clients remove their dentures at night, which allows the gum tissue to rest. It is important to ensure that they have a container of cleaning solution or water for soaking the dentures. Make sure that the dentures fit well. Loose-fitting dentures can make it difficult to eat. Be sensitive when helping with dentures, and remember that some clients may be embarrassed to be seen without their dentures.

Record daily dental care for each client.

Mouth/Oral Care

If the client is not taking food and drink, their mouth can be become dry and cracked. Check the mouth for sores and attend to mouth care regularly. Use a lubricant to keep lips moisturised.

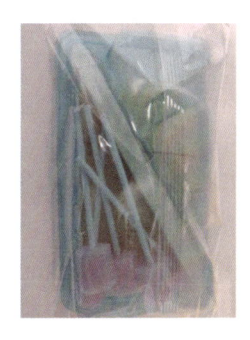

Foam swabs can be used to hydrate the mouth. Care must be taken if using foam swabs, so that the client does not bite down and break the foam head off, which will lead to the risk of choking. Foam swabs should only be used if the client is assessed as being suitable and not at risk of biting down on the swab. Mouth cleansers can be used safely instead of foam swabs. They gently clean the mouth and teeth and are designed to fit safely in the mouth, without the risk of choking.

Shaving

Men may need assistance with shaving or they may only need access to shaving facilities.

Task

You are asked to shave a client. He is 92 years old and his name is Peter. His hands are unsteady and weak, and he is unable to help you with the task.

Describe step by step how you will shave Peter.

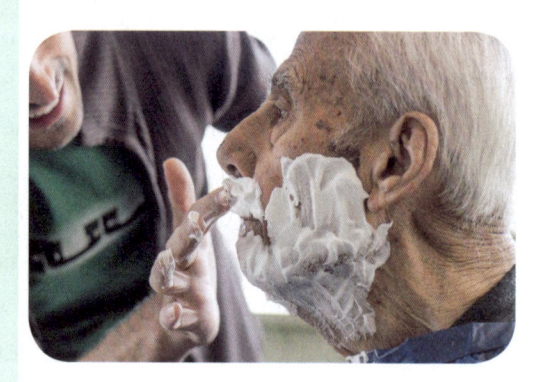

Older women and **facial hair**: some older women can have a good deal of facial hair and may feel embarrassed by this. Ask them how they normally deal with it, e.g. using a depilatory cream. Assist them with this if necessary.

Hand Care and Foot Care

Ensure that the client's fingernails are clean – you can soak the hands in warm water and clean the nails gently. Moisturise the hands.

For foot care, soak the feet, wash carefully between the toes, dry carefully and thoroughly and clean the nails. Moisturise the feet. A client's toenails should only be cut by a chiropodist.

CHAPTER 06: GROOMING, DRESSING AND SENSORY NEEDS

Look out for any problems with the hands and feet, such as sores or fungal infections. Report any concerns to your supervisor or nurse in charge.

Make-up

Your client may like to wear make-up, and this may be part of their daily routine. Wearing make-up can be part of their identity and will contribute to a positive self-image, making them feel good about themselves. Make sure that they have access to any products or equipment needed, including a mirror.

Ask them what assistance they need. Remember, you don't need to have the skills of a make-up artist to help an individual with their make-up.

Cultural Considerations

Check with your client how they wish to attend to their grooming. Some ethnic groups may have different rituals when attending to the grooming of their hair, due to different hair types. The hair may have a coarse texture and oils may be used to maintain it. Ask your client how they attend to their grooming.

> **Task** Identify some cultural preferences in relation to grooming that you might encounter.

DRESSING

Clean underwear and clothing should be worn each day, and if food spills occur during the day clothes should be changed immediately. Family should be informed when clothing needs to be replaced or purchased.

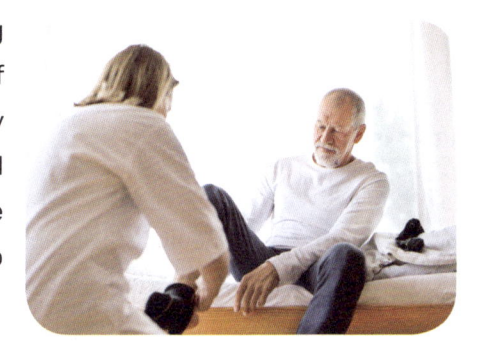

COMPLETE CARE SKILLS

Assist the client with dressing. Many care settings encourage their clients and residents to get up and dress every day. It helps to give them a structured routine. Even if you are working as a carer in a hospital setting, looking after acutely ill people, many of them will still be able to get out of bed and dress during the day. We can feel vulnerable and helpless if we are meeting people in our nightclothes. It will improve how we feel about ourselves if we are dressed.

#EndPJParalysis

#EndPJParalysis is a global social movement, embraced by nurses, therapists and medical colleagues, that aims to get patients up, dressed and moving.

Having patients in their day clothes while in hospital, rather than in pyjamas (PJs) or gowns, enhances dignity, autonomy and, in many instances, shortens their length of stay. For patients over the age of 80, a week in bed can lead to ten years of muscle ageing, 1.5 kg of muscle loss, and may lead to increased dependency and demotivation. Getting patients up and moving has been shown to reduce falls, improve patient experience and reduce length of stay by up to 1.5 days.

#EndPJParalysis puts the focus on quality of patient time and experience. It asks the question, 'If you had 1,000 days to live, would you like to spend them in hospital?' (www.endpjparalysis.com/)

Points to Remember

- Give choices. Ask 'What would you like to wear today?' If the client has difficulty making choices, e.g. if they have Alzheimer's disease, limit the choices by asking, 'Would you like to wear the red top or the blue one today?'

CHAPTER 06: GROOMING, DRESSING AND SENSORY NEEDS

- Assist as necessary with putting the clothes on.
- Never rush the client.
- Encourage independence by letting the client do as much as possible themselves.

In some cases, you may need to recommend certain clothing to the client; for example, elasticated skirts and pants, loose-fitting tops with buttons at the neck, and front-opening clothes are easier for the client to manage themselves. Footwear should be safe and include Velcro fastening or elasticated shoe-laces which make it easier for the client to put the footwear on.

Using dressing aids can encourage the client to dress themselves, e.g. long shoe horns, aids for putting socks or stockings on, zip pullers, grabbers and coat reachers support independence.

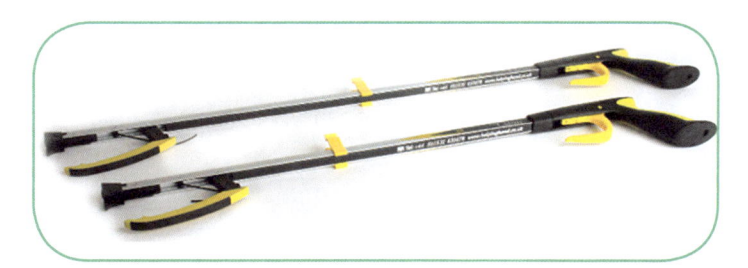

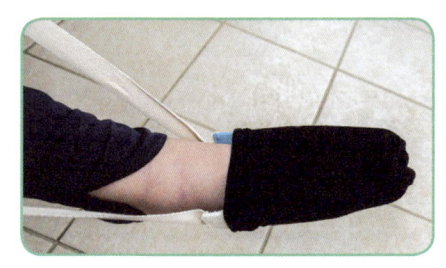

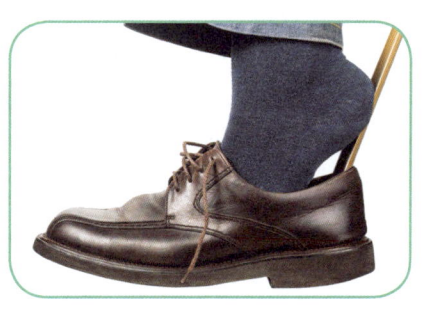

Task Research the aids that can be used to help with dressing.

The client may have had help with using these aids from the occupational therapist, but you may have to remind them about how to use them. This may take longer than dressing them, but it is important to encourage independence.

Some clients have certain clothes that form a part of their self-identity. Some older men like to wear braces or peaked caps in bed. Some clients will also want to wear their jewellery. Respect the client's choices and their individuality.

Compliment the client on how they look. We all like to be told that we look nice. This will promote a positive self-image.

Cultural Considerations

The client may dress in traditional clothing. Clients from Pakistan often wear a shalwar kameez. This is worn by men and women and consists of a long tunic worn over loose trousers. Women from India may wish to wear a sari. Some women from other countries may wear a veil. Give assistance with their clothing as necessary.

Revision Questions:

1. Why is it important to ensure that a client attends to their grooming?
2. How can you promote positive self-image through helping with grooming?
3. Why is foot care important?

Key words/phrases:

mouth care

hand care

foot care

MEETING NUTRITIONAL NEEDS 07

The person you are caring for may need assistance with eating and drinking. Good nutrition and hydration leads to good health and promotes well-being. It can help to prevent disease and sickness, promote healing and recovery if we are already sick and it can also influence our mood. Eating and drinking can be a social activity as we usually eat at set times and with others. However, some individuals are not able to look after their own nutritional needs and may require help to eat and drink.

IN THIS CHAPTER YOU WILL LEARN ABOUT:

- The elements of a balanced diet
- How to help an individual to eat and drink
- Aids that can help a client with eating and drinking
- The importance of promoting respect and dignity
- Special dietary considerations
- The importance of recording what the person has eaten and drunk

NUTRITION

The carer should have some knowledge and understanding about healthy eating and drinking. Our diet needs to be balanced and varied. Some animals only need to eat one type of food (e.g. cows only need grass) and the animal's system is then able to make all the other nutrients needed for the healthy functioning of the animal. Humans cannot make all the nutrients needed, so we must get them from food. It is important that we eat a varied diet, to ensure that we are getting all the nutrients we need. Deficiency in any nutrient can lead to illness and health problems.

THE FOOD PYRAMID

The food pyramid is a visual guide for understanding which foods we should eat, and in what proportions. It's a guide for the whole population from the age of five years and upwards. We should eat foods from all food groups and in the correct portion sizes and amounts.

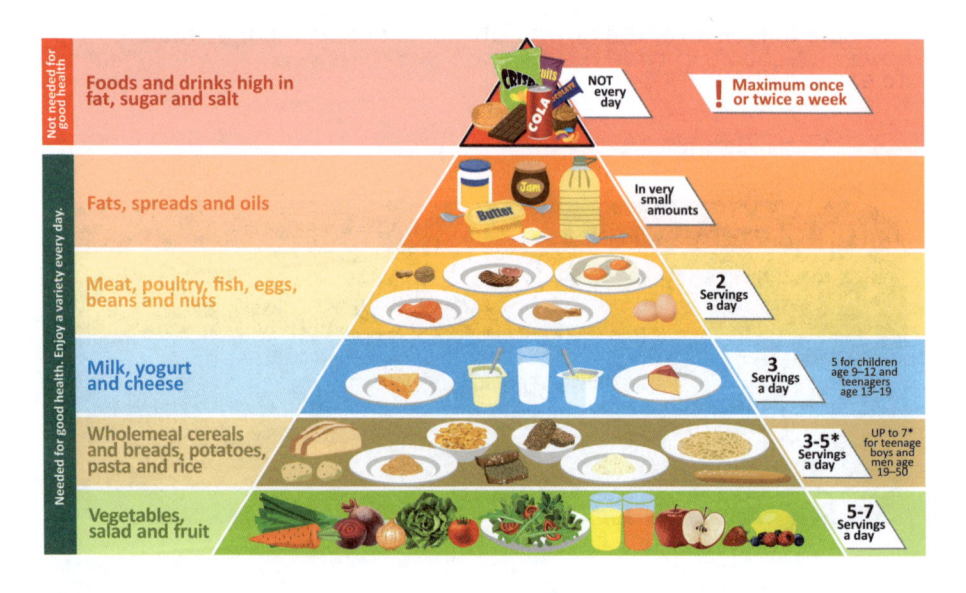

Not needed for good health	Foods and drinks high in fat, sugar and salt	NOT every day — Maximum once or twice a week
Needed for good health. Enjoy a variety every day.	Fats, spreads and oils	In very small amounts
	Meat, poultry, fish, eggs, beans and nuts	2 Servings a day
	Milk, yogurt and cheese	3 Servings a day — 5 for children age 9–12 and teenagers age 13–19
	Wholemeal cereals and breads, potatoes, pasta and rice	3-5* Servings a day — UP to 7* for teenage boys and men age 19–50
	Vegetables, salad and fruit	5-7 Servings a day

Task: Write down everything you ate yesterday. How does it compare with the recommendations of the food pyramid?

The food we eat is categorised according to the main nutrient that the food provides. The main types are: carbohydrates, proteins, fats, vitamins and minerals. Water, although not classed as a nutrient, is also essential for life.

Carbohydrates

The main function of carbohydrates is to provide energy, which we need to maintain the basic functions of the body. We also need energy for all our daily activities. In Ireland we get most of our carbohydrates from potatoes, rice, pasta and bread. We should choose healthy carbohydrates such as wholemeal or wholegrain bread, brown rice or pasta, as they contain fibre, which is essential for a healthy digestive system. Unhealthy carbohydrates that are high in sugar, such as cakes and biscuits, should be avoided or limited to once a week.

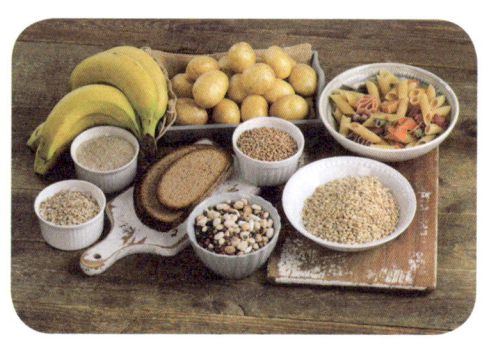

Protein

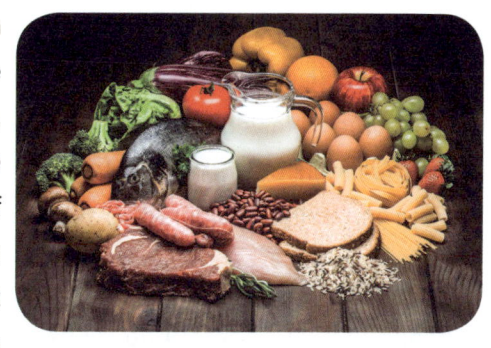

Protein is needed for growth and repair and can also be used for energy. Muscles, organs and the immune system are mostly made up of protein. The body uses protein to make haemoglobin, the part of red blood cells that carries oxygen to every part of the body. We get proteins from animal and plant sources. Meat, poultry, fish and eggs are good sources of animal protein; soya beans, nuts, lentils, peas and cereals are good sources of plant protein.

Fat

This is an essential nutrient that is needed for energy. This energy can be stored in the body. Fat gives shape to the body; it cushions our skin and protects us; and it acts as insulation against heat loss and keeps us warm. It covers our nerve cells, insulating them and making them work more efficiently, and acts as a shock absorber that protects the organs. Fats in our diet are an important source of fat-soluble vitamins (vitamins A, D, E and K). Fats form part of every cell membrane.

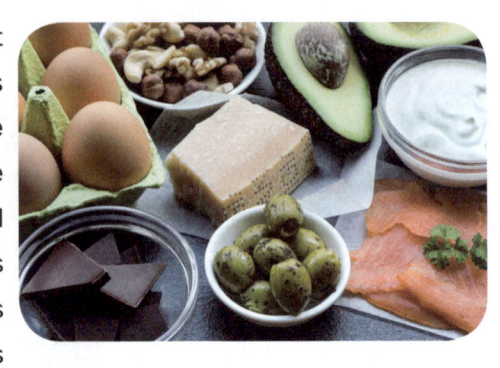

Some fatty acids, such as omega 3 and 6, are essential. This means that the body cannot make them and we have to obtain them from our diet. The essential fatty acids are very important for good health and have been linked to many health benefits.

Fats in food are either saturated or unsaturated. Saturated fats are found in meat, meat products and dairy products. Unsaturated fats mostly come from vegetable sources (sunflower oil, olive oil, soya oil) or oily fish (salmon, trout, mackerel, etc.) and soft margarines. Unsaturated fats are generally considered better for us than saturated fats.

Too much fat or too much of the wrong type of fat in the diet can lead to health problems, contribute to heart disease, higher blood pressure and cholesterol levels and obesity.

Vitamins and Minerals

Vitamins and minerals have very important functions in the body, and prolonged deficiencies can lead to health problems. They are found in the foods we eat. The main vitamins are A, B, C, D, E and K.

Water-soluble Vitamins

Water-soluble vitamins cannot be stored in our bodies and are readily excreted. These include vitamins B_1, B_2, B_3, B_6, B_9 (folate or folic acid), B_{12} and C.

Nutrient	Function	Sources
Vitamin B_1 (thiamine)	Releases energy from carbohydrate. It is also involved in the functioning of the nervous system and the heart.	Whole grains, nuts, meat (especially pork), fruit and vegetables, fortified breakfast cereals.
Vitamin B_2 (riboflavin)	Releases energy from carbohydrate, protein and fat. It is also involved in the transport and metabolism of iron in the body and is needed for the normal structure and functioning of the skin and linings of the organs.	Milk, eggs, rice, fortified breakfast cereals, liver, legumes, mushrooms, green vegetables.
Vitamin B_3 (niacin)	Releases energy from food, and is important for the normal structure of the skin and organ linings. It also keeps the digestive and nervous systems healthy.	Meat, wheat and maize flour, eggs, dairy products, yeast.

Nutrient	Function	Sources
Vitamin B$_6$	Involved in the use of protein, and helps to form haemoglobin in blood (the substance that carries oxygen around the body).	Poultry, white fish, milk, eggs, whole grains, soya beans, peanuts, some vegetables.
Vitamin B$_9$ (folate/folic acid)	Needed for the formation of healthy red blood cells, for the nervous system and specifically for the development of the nervous system in unborn babies.	Green leafy vegetables, brown rice, peas, oranges, bananas, fortified breakfast cereals.
Vitamin B$_{12}$	Important for making red blood cells and to keep the nervous system healthy. Also helps to release energy from food.	Meat, fish, milk, cheese, eggs, yeast extract and fortified breakfast cereals.
Vitamin C	Acts as an antioxidant and is important for the normal structure and functioning of body tissues. It also helps the body to absorb iron from non-meat sources such as vegetables, as well as assisting the healing process.	Fresh fruits, especially citrus fruits and berries; green vegetables, peppers and tomatoes. Also found in potatoes (especially new potatoes).

Fat-soluble Vitamins

Fat-soluble vitamins are absorbed through the gut with the help of fat. They include vitamins A, D, E and K.

Nutrient	Functions	Sources
Vitamin A	Important for the normal structure and functioning of the skin and organ linings, e.g. in the lungs. It also helps with vision in dim light as well as keeping the immune system healthy.	Liver, whole milk, cheese, butter, margarine, carrots, dark green leafy vegetables and orange-coloured fruits, e.g. mangoes and apricots.
Vitamin D	Needed for the absorption of calcium and phosphorus from foods, to keep bones healthy. Recent research also suggests that vitamin D enhances immune function and improves muscle strength.	Oily fish, eggs, fortified cereals, margarine. Most is obtained through the action of sunlight on our skin during the summer months.
Vitamin E	Acts as an antioxidant and protects the cells in our bodies against damage.	Vegetable oils, nuts and seeds.
Vitamin K	Needed for the normal clotting of blood and for normal bone structure.	Green leafy vegetables, meat and dairy products.

Source: British Nutrition Foundation.

Minerals

The body uses minerals to perform many different functions, from building strong bones to transmitting nerve impulses. Some minerals are even used to make hormones or maintain a normal heartbeat. The main minerals in our diet are:

Nutrient	Function	Sources
Calcium	Important for the formation and maintenance of strong bones and teeth, as well as the functioning of nerves and muscles. It is also involved in blood clotting.	Milk, cheese and other dairy products, some green leafy vegetables such as broccoli, fortified soya bean products, bread.
Fluoride	Helps with the formation of strong teeth and protects against dental decay (caries).	Fluoridated water, tea, fish, toothpaste.
Iodine	Needed to make thyroid hormones, which control many metabolic processes, and keep our bodies healthy.	Milk, sea fish, shellfish, seaweed and iodine-fortified foods, such as some salt.

Nutrient	Function	Sources
Iron	Required for making red blood cells, which transport oxygen around the body. Also needed for normal metabolism and the functioning of enzymes that remove unwanted substances from the body.	Liver, red meat, pulses, nuts, eggs, dried fruits, poultry, fish, whole grains, dark green leafy vegetables.
Magnesium	Needed for the release of energy from food and to maintain water balance. It is also important for the formation of strong muscles, bones and teeth.	Found widely in foods, particularly green leafy vegetables, nuts, bread, fish, meat, dairy products.
Phosphorous	Needed for the formation of healthy bones and teeth, and for the release of energy from food.	Red meat, dairy products, fish, poultry, bread, rice, oats.
Potassium	Controls water balance in our bodies and helps maintain a healthy blood pressure. It is also involved in the normal functioning of nerves.	Fruit (especially bananas), vegetables, meat, fish, shellfish, milk, nuts, seeds, pulses.

Nutrient	Function	Sources
Selenium	An important component of the body's defence system that protects our bodies against damage. It is also necessary for the use of iodine in thyroid hormone production, as well as the normal functioning of the reproductive system.	Brazil nuts, bread, fish, meat, eggs.
Sodium	Helps regulate the water content in the body and the balance of electrolytes. Also involved in the use of energy, as well as the functioning of the central nervous system.	Very small amounts in raw foods. Often added during processing, preparation, preservation and serving. Currently intakes of sodium are too high and so although some sodium is essential, most people need to reduce their intake substantially.
Zinc	Required for the use of carbohydrate, protein and fat. Needed for cell division, growth and tissue repair. Also necessary for normal reproductive development, the immune system and healing of wounds.	Meat, milk, cheese, eggs, shellfish, wholegrain cereals, nuts and pulses.

Source: British Nutrition Foundation

Water

Fluids are essential for our health. Water is essential for life and although humans can survive for a number of weeks without food, they cannot go without fluids for more than two to three days. Water makes up about 60% of the body and is used in all cells, organs and tissues to help regulate temperature and maintain other bodily functions. It acts as a lubricant for joints and eyes. It is the main component of saliva, which helps us swallow. It provides the medium in which most reactions in the body occur, acts as a cushion for the nervous system and helps get rid of waste.

Water helps regulate body temperature and is lost from the body through breathing, sweating and urination. The body cannot produce enough water to meet all its needs, so most of the water we need must be provided by our food and drink. If we do not consume enough water, we become dehydrated. It is important to rehydrate by drinking fluids and eating foods that contain water. The amount of fluid we need depends on how active we are and how warm it is. To stay healthy we should drink about eight glasses or 1.2 litres per day.

The body loses fluids through vigorous exercise, sweat in high heat, fever or an illness that causes vomiting or diarrhoea. It is important to increase your fluid intake if fluid is lost for any of these reasons so that you can restore your body's natural hydration levels.

ASSISTING A CLIENT AT MEALTIMES

Planning

Before you help a client, you need to know what they can or cannot eat or if they have special dietary needs such as a modified/textured diet. You need to know if they can assist themselves or if they need assistance from a carer and, if so, how much assistance is needed. You will also need to know if it is safe for the client to eat, as some clients may be at risk of choking and may have special requirements. You may need to be trained in assisting these clients with their nutritional needs.

Adapt the level of assistance needed according to the client. The client may only need you to cut the food or slice the bread, or they may need full assistance. Consult their care plan to determine the level of assistance needed and any likes or dislikes the client has. Consult with the nurse in charge or supervisor and also ask the client what help they need and what they like to eat.

Preparation

+ **Prepare yourself:** Attend to hand hygiene first. Wear PPE as appropriate and according to the policies of your workplace. Aprons worn for hygiene purposes should be removed and a clean apron put on. In some settings the aprons are colour-coded according to the task. This acts as a reminder to change your apron.

+ **Prepare the client:** Introduce yourself ('Hello, my name is ...'). Gain consent and give explanations and choices. The client should have control over what they eat every day. In many care settings clients eat in a communal dining room. Assist the client to the dining room. Ask the client first if they wish to eat in the dining area – some clients may prefer to eat on their own. If they prefer to eat in their room, sit them out of bed. If they are unable to sit out, sit them up in the bed, well supported by pillows. It is easier to eat if you are upright. Allow the client to wash their hands before eating and make sure they have a napkin before you start. Clothing protectors are sometimes used in some settings. If the client is an adult, this can be seen as treating them like a child, but some adult clients like to use a clothing protector in case of spillages. The consent of the client is the most important thing.

- **Prepare the environment:** Clear the area and remove any offensive objects such as urinals, sputum pots, etc. Ensure the table is clean. Non-slip mats may be useful to place the plates on. If you are assisting the client to eat, sit in a chair; don't stand over the client as this may make them feel intimidated. It is better to sit at eye level.

Points to Remember when Assisting at Mealtimes

- Remember the dignity of the client when you are helping them to eat.
- Encourage independence.
- Some clients only need supervision or reminding to eat.
- Make sure the food is at the correct temperature.
- The food should be presented in an attractive way.
- Make sure the patient has a napkin to protect their clothes.
- Cut the food if necessary.
- If the client wears dentures, ensure they are in place.
- Do not hurry the client – let them eat at their own speed.
- Allow the client to swallow the food before offering another mouthful.
- Respect the client's dignity and use the napkin to wipe dribbles.
- Encourage them to eat and drink but do not force them.
- Don't forget to help with fluids. Older clients may forget to drink if not reminded.
- In some cases, a thickener may need to be added to fluids to reduce the risk of choking. Follow your workplace guidelines when using thickeners.

> + Use any feeding aids that will help the client, such as a non-slip mat, plate guards, plate dividers, eating utensils with adapted handles, cups and beakers with lids.
>
> + Monitor for any signs of a decrease in the person's ability to swallow (signs of aspiration).

Aids for Assisting at Mealtimes

A wide variety of utensils can be used to help a client to eat and drink safely and independently.

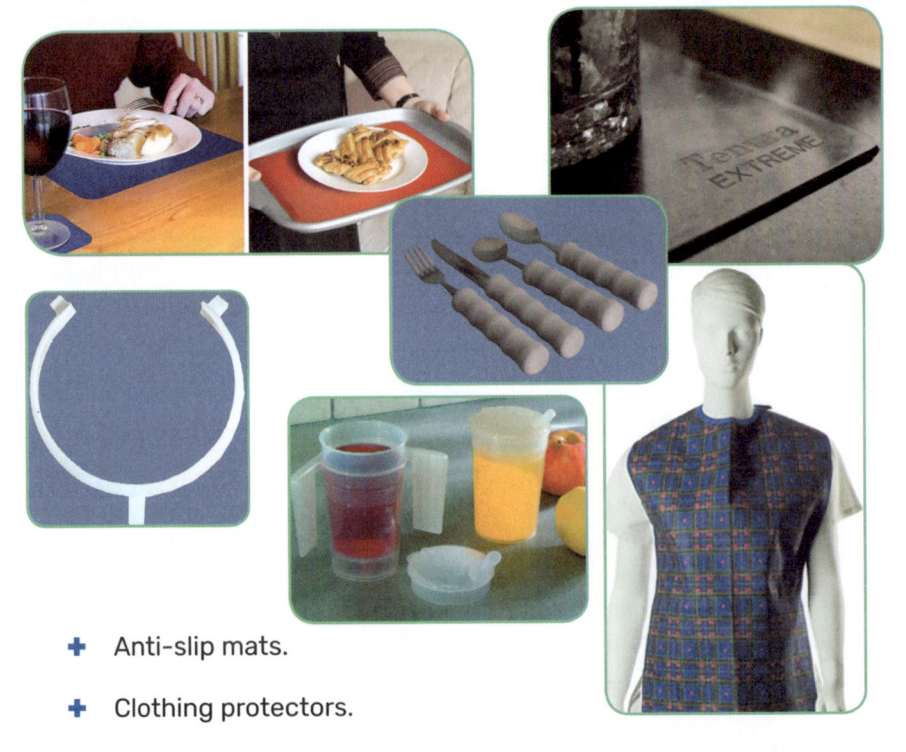

+ Anti-slip mats.

+ Clothing protectors.

+ Beakers with a lid to prevent spillages. The cups can be two-handled to make them easier to hold.

+ Plate guards can be used to make it easier for the client to scoop up their food.

+ Special cutlery with foam handles make it easier to hold.

CHAPTER 07: MEETING NUTRITIONAL NEEDS

Task Research the different types of feeding aids and how they are used. If you are in a workplace, what types of feeding aids are used in your workplace?

Task In pairs, feed each other a yoghurt. Then give each other a drink.
How did you feel feeding another adult? How did you feel being fed?

SPECIAL DIETARY REQUIREMENTS

Your client may have to eat a special diet.

Modified/Textured Diet

Some clients must have their food puréed. The meal should not be puréed all together as this creates an unappetising brown mush. The foods should be puréed separately and placed separately on the plate.

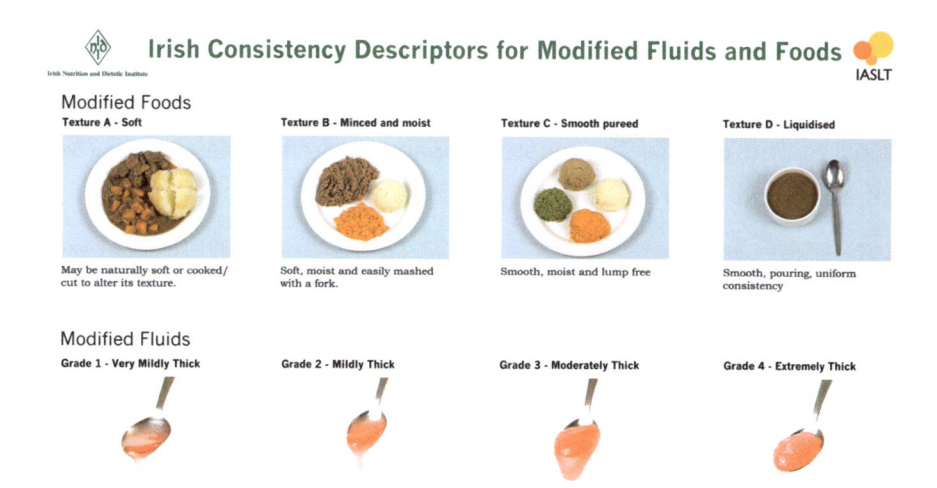

Irish Consistency Descriptors for Modified Fluids and Foods

Modified Foods

- **Texture A - Soft**: May be naturally soft or cooked/cut to alter its texture.
- **Texture B - Minced and moist**: Soft, moist and easily mashed with a fork.
- **Texture C - Smooth puréed**: Smooth, moist and lump free
- **Texture D - Liquidised**: Smooth, pouring, uniform consistency

Modified Fluids

- Grade 1 - Very Mildly Thick
- Grade 2 - Mildly Thick
- Grade 3 - Moderately Thick
- Grade 4 - Extremely Thick

Courtesy of IASLT & the HSE. More information can be found at www.iddsi.org

Diabetes

This is a condition in which the body is not able to control the blood sugars, resulting in high blood sugar levels. People who live with diabetes can eat a wide and varied diet, which should follow healthy eating guidelines. Fatty foods and sugary treats should be avoided or taken in small amounts. Water is the recommended drink, although tea and coffee can also be taken. Special diabetic foods are not recommended as they are often high in fats and calories. As a carer it is important to check that the client is eating and not skipping meals. (See Diabetes Ireland, www.diabetes.ie.)

Coeliac Disease

A client with coeliac disease must eat a gluten-free diet. (Gluten is a protein found in cereals – wheat, rye, barley and oats.) Gluten can cause damage to the intestinal wall, resulting in stomach cramping, diarrhoea or constipation. There is no cure, so someone with coeliac disease must avoid gluten for their lifetime. Check to ensure that the foods they are eating are gluten-free. It is important to prepare meals for coeliac clients separately, using separate utensils, condiments and spreads to avoid cross-contamination. Remember, a single crumb is enough to cause a bad reaction. Always ensure that the food for people with coeliac disease is prepared separately from other foods. (See Coeliac Society of Ireland, www.coeliac.ie.)

Cystic Fibrosis

This is a condition in which the lining of body tissues produces a sticky mucus. When too much mucus is produced by the lining of the intestinal wall it can block the absorption of nutrients. People living with cystic fibrosis need a high-calorie, high-fat diet. They also need salt in their diet as they tend to lose salt through excess sweating. (See Cystic Fibrosis Ireland, www.cfireland.ie.)

Lactose Intolerance

A person with lactose intolerance has difficulty breaking down lactose in foods. Lactose is a sugar found in dairy products. Check with the client how they manage their condition: some people who are lactose intolerant can eat dairy products in small amounts; others are advised to eat a lactose-free diet. Medicines are available to treat the condition, some of which come in a liquid form to be added to milk, while others can be chewed before a meal or a snack. As dairy is an essential source of calcium, necessary for strong bones, it must be replaced with other calcium-rich foods if it is omitted from the client's diet.

Nut Allergies

Be aware of any nut allergies in the care setting and take appropriate action to ensure that no nuts of any kind are introduced into the environment. Clients with nut allergies can be prone to severe reactions, resulting in life-or-death situations. Check with the client's care plan or your supervisor with regard to action to be taken if there is any allergic reaction.

Vegetarian and Vegan Diets

Clients opting for a vegetarian diet avoid eating meat, fish or poultry. A vegetarian diet consisting of plant-based foods, diary products and eggs provides all essential nutrients in the diet.

Vegans have a more restricted diet as they avoid all foods that come from an animal source, such as meat, dairy, eggs and honey. The vegan diet can also provide all the essential nutrients needed, although there is a risk of deficiencies in nutrients that are mostly found in foods from an animal source, such as calcium and vitamin B12. They may have to take supplements to replace the vitamins and minerals absent from the diet.

CULTURAL CONSIDERATIONS

Religion and ethnicity influence our diet. In the past Catholics did not eat meat on Fridays, and some people continue to observe this tradition. Jewish people eat kosher foods and Muslims eat halal meat. Neither Muslims nor Jews eat pork. Muslims observe a period of fasting during Ramadan. Hindus believe that the cow is sacred and don't eat beef. Many Hindus are vegetarian. People from different ethnic backgrounds may prefer different types of food, such as spicy food. Choice of diet should be offered to clients.

AFTER MEALTIME

Clear away the utensils and replace any of the client's belongings that you moved before the meal. Allow the client to wash their hands and ensure that the face is clean and free from dribbles or spilled food. If clothing is food-stained, assist the client to change.

Safely remove any PPE and attend to your own hand hygiene.

RECORDING AND REPORTING

You may need to record what the client has eaten and drunk. Records to be kept are Food Intake Charts (see Appendix 1), which detail everything the client has eaten; and Fluid Balance Chart (fluid intake and output) (see Appendix 2), which record all fluids, including amounts, consumed by the client.

Report any developments or changes in the client's food intake to your supervisor or nurse.

Exercise:

Mary is 84 years old. She has fractured both her arms following a fall down a flight of stairs. She is normally independent and healthy but now both arms are in a cast and she is unable to feed herself. She has recently been diagnosed with diabetes.

+ Discuss how you will help Mary to eat and drink.

Hint: Remember the checklist: plan and prepare, assist with mealtimes, tidy up afterwards, record and report.

Revision Questions:

1. What are the main food groups?
2. Name three foods from each group.
3. Why is water intake so important?
4. List three special dietary considerations and explain how you would accommodate each diet.
5. How can you ensure that the client's dignity is maintained when you assist with mealtimes?

Key words/phrases:

- food pyramid
- carbohydrates
- proteins
- fats
- vitamins and minerals
- water
- Fluid Balance Chart (fluid intake and output)
- special dietary considerations
- soft diet
- coeliac disease
- lactose intolerance
- nut allergy
- diabetes

CONTINENCE PROMOTION AND TOILETING

08

We take for granted many of the things we do every day. When we get up in the morning one of the first things we do is go to the toilet. Throughout the day, we will make many more visits to the toilet. Some clients may be unable to do this independently and will need your assistance. Using the toilet is a very personal thing, and needing assistance with toileting can be very embarrassing. In this chapter we will look at the kind of assistance needed by your clients and the ways in which you can help them.

IN THIS CHAPTER YOU WILL LEARN ABOUT:

- The different levels of assistance needed
- The importance of maintaining respect and dignity when assisting with toileting needs
- The different types of care equipment used
- How to assist a person with their toileting needs
- Various aids to toileting: commode, bedpan, urinal, sluice room, incontinence pad, catheter, stoma bag
- How to assist a person who is incontinent, and ways of promoting continence
- Being aware of individual needs, including cultural considerations

IDENTIFYING THE LEVEL OF ASSISTANCE NEEDED

Many clients will need some level of assistance with their toileting needs. In many cases, minimal assistance is needed, and you will only be required to:

- Remind them to go the toilet
- Walk them to the toilet and supervise their toileting needs
- Wheel them in a wheelchair to the toilet and assist them to transfer
- Assist with bedpans or commodes
- Assist with incontinence wear.

When assisting with toileting needs, try wherever possible to bring clients to the bathroom to attend to their toileting needs, as it is more private and allows the client to maintain their dignity.

TOILETING AIDS

- **Commodes** are portable toilets and can be used by the client's bedside if they have difficulty mobilising to the toilet.
- **Bedpans** can be used for clients who are unable to get out of bed.
- **Urinals** can be used by men for passing urine. It is also possible to use female urinals, which are shaped for the female anatomy.
- Clients who are incontinent may have to wear **incontinence pads**.

Using a Commode or a Bedpan

If a client is not able to go to the bathroom to attend to their toileting needs, they may require a commode beside their bed, or they may need to use a bedpan.

A commode is a portable toilet chair – some have wheels. A commode allows a client to go to the toilet in locations other than the bathroom, typically by the bedside. If a client requires a commode, you need to plan and prepare before assisting them.

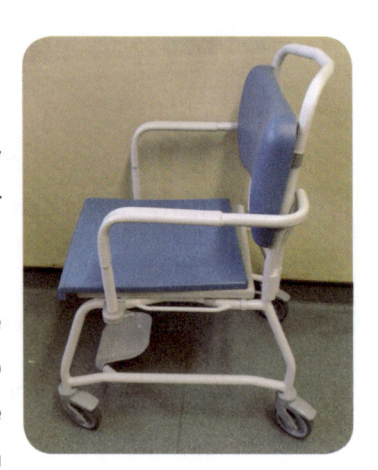

- **Plan:** Check the care plan and the client's notes, which will indicate what kind of assistance is needed. Determine whether two carers are needed and speak to the nurse in charge or your supervisor to see if there are any special circumstances to be considered. Check to see if a hoist is needed. Talk to the client and find out what assistance is needed.

- **Prepare yourself:** Attend to hand hygiene and wear PPE (disposable apron and disposable gloves).

- **Prepare the client:** Introduce yourself ('Hello, my name is …'), give explanations and gain consent. Speak to the client in words that they understand. People use many different words for urine and faeces and some older clients may also use different words for the commode and bedpan; for example, an older person might ask you to bring them the pot.

- **Prepare the environment:** Close any curtains and doors. Ask visitors to leave. Move furniture if necessary. Get equipment needed – the commode, toilet paper, wipes for cleaning the client's hands afterwards. A hoist may be needed to transfer the client to the commode.

Helping the Client Use the Commode

Promote independence by encouraging the client to see to their own needs where possible. Place the commode close to the client – the distance will depend on the client's level of mobility. Make sure that the wheel brakes of the commode are on. Remove the lid of the commode. Assist the client as necessary to stand, assist them with their clothing, and help them to lower on to the commode seat. If the client is safe to be left unattended, make sure that they have access to the nurse-call button. Respect the client's privacy. When the client has used the toilet, assist to wipe as necessary. Help them to stand and pull their clothes back up. Assist them back to their chair or to the bed. Allow them to clean their hands. Place the lid on the commode. Knock off the brakes and wheel the commode to the sluice room for safe disposal of the contents.

> Nursing homes and hospitals have a room called a sluice room, which is a room for disposing of toilet waste. It will have facilities for cleaning the toileting equipment. The contents of the commode should be safely disposed of, and the commode bucket should be placed in the bedpan washer, a machine for cleaning and disinfecting commode buckets, bedpans and urinals.

Clean the commode as per the policies and protocols in your workplace. In nursing homes, a client who needs a commode has their own commode assigned to them for their use only. Return the cleaned commode to its storage place.

When you have finished assisting the client, remove and safely dispose of PPE. Attend to hand hygiene.

Using Bedpans and Urinal Bottles

Some clients are unable to get out of bed to go to the bathroom. They may use a bedpan or a urinal. Urinal bottles are mostly used by male clients, although specially shaped female urinal bottles are available. The client passes urine into the urinal bottle.

Bedpans are placed under the client in bed and they pass urine or open their bowels on the bedpan.

When a client needs to use a bedpan or urinal bottle, plan and prepare as for using a commode. Ensure the dignity and respect of the client is maintained. Two carers may be needed to assist the client on the bedpan.

The client may be able to lift themselves on to the bedpan. If they can't, you may have to ask them to roll to one side, position the bedpan under them, then assist them to roll back onto the bedpan.

Keep the client covered when they are using the bedpan or urinal. Afterwards, help them wipe themselves. Allow the client to clean their hands after use. Safely dispose of the waste in the sluice room. Place the bedpan or urinal bottle into the bedpan washer. Store the bedpan/urinal safely afterwards.

Remove and safely dispose of PPE. Attend to your own hand hygiene.

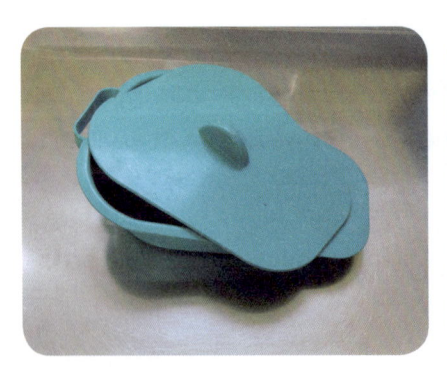

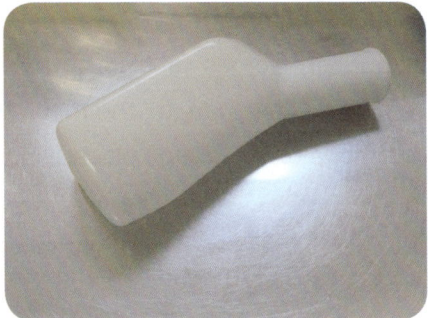

INCONTINENCE

Clients who are incontinent are unable to control the passing of urine or faeces. Some clients who are incontinent wear incontinence pads, and the carer will have to assist the client to change the pads.

Points to Consider when Caring for an Incontinent Client

Check the client regularly to make sure that they are not wet or soiled. This may be embarrassing for the client and their relatives, and they may not be able to tell you that they are soiled. If a client is left too long in a wet and soiled incontinence pad, it can lead to sore skin and it increases their risk of getting a pressure sore.

Select the most suitable incontinence wear – they come in different sizes and types.

> **Task** What types of incontinence wear are used in your workplace?

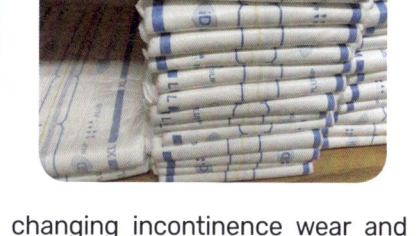

Wear PPE (gloves and aprons) when changing incontinence wear and attend to hand hygiene before and after. Dispose of used incontinence pads safely. Clean the client with warm soapy water and then dry the client.

Promoting Continence

Some people you may be caring for avoid drinking because they have a fear of incontinence or are worried that they won't make it to the toilet in time. However, it's important for a healthy bladder that we drink plenty of fluids, the recommended amount being six to eight glasses of fluid a day. This doesn't have to be just water – milk or fruit juices are also good choices. Tea, coffee and fizzy drinks may irritate the bladder.

For healthy stools, it is recommended that we eat plenty of fibre to prevent constipation. Staying as active and mobile as possible will also help prevent constipation.

The HSE suggests the following tips for managing incontinence:

- Good personal hygiene decreases the risk of skin problems and unpleasant odours.
- Keep a commode or urine bottle beside the bed at night.
- Remember to use the toilet regularly.
- Wear clothes that are easy to undo or remove.
- Ensure that the toilet is easy to get to.
- When necessary, wear appropriate absorbent underwear (HSE 'Continence Promotion').

Catheter Care

Some of your clients may have a urinary catheter in place. This is a tube that is inserted into the bladder and held in place by an inflated balloon. The tube is attached to a bag. Urine from the bladder goes directly into the external bag. The catheter bag will need to be emptied into a jug. Ensure that good hygiene standards are maintained when emptying the catheter bag. Measure and record the amount of urine.

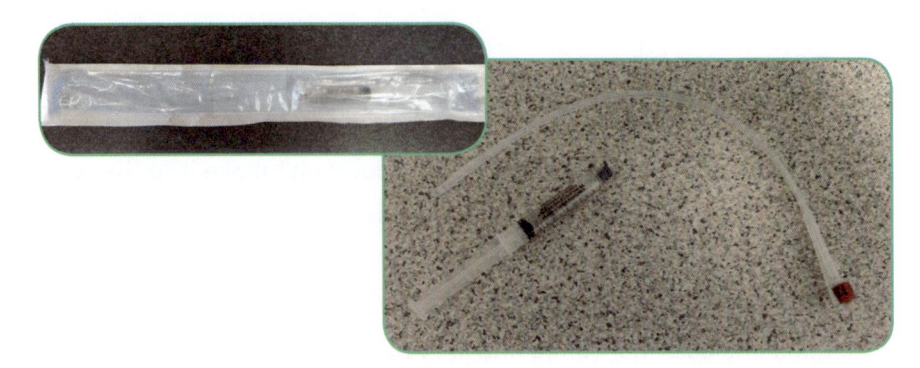

Stoma Care

A stoma is a surgically created opening on the outside of the abdomen. The faeces leaves the body through this opening, rather than by the anus. A bag is placed over the stoma to collect the faeces. The carer may have to assist the client with care of the stoma by either emptying the stoma bag or changing the bag. If you have not cared for someone with a stoma before, you will be shown in your workplace how to care for the stoma. The client may feel embarrassed and uncomfortable because of the stoma. Never express disgust when caring for someone with a stoma.

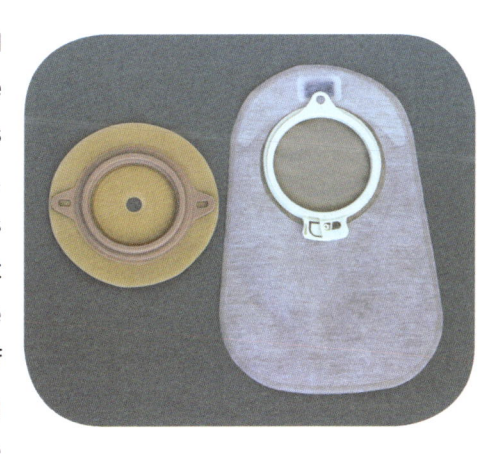

DIGNITY AND RESPECT

When assisting another person with their toileting needs, it is very important to maintain their respect and dignity. Our toileting needs are very private, and many clients will feel very embarrassed and apologetic about their needs.

- Always be discreet when asking a client about their toileting needs – speak quietly.
- Use language that the client is familiar with.
- Where possible, keep the client covered, and don't expose them more than is necessary.
- Ensure privacy. Where possible, bring the client to the bathroom rather than using a bedpan or a commode. Remember that in

shared spaces a curtain pulled around a client doesn't give them full privacy.

+ Never express disgust when assisting a client with toileting.

CULTURAL CONSIDERATIONS

Some religious or ethnic groups may prefer to have someone of their own gender assist them with toileting needs. People of some religions wash after toileting, both defecating and urinating. In the West we tend to use toilet paper first and then wash. Disposable cups should be made available in bathrooms to facilitate this practice. In the Muslim faith, the left hand is generally used for any washing conducted after toileting.

RECORDING AND REPORTING

You may need to record whether the client opened their bowels. You may need to measure and record any urine output on a **Fluid Balance Chart (fluid intake and output)** (see Appendix 2). If you notice anything unusual, this needs to be reported orally to your supervisor, and recorded in the client's daily care plan. Use the Bristol Stool Chart when reporting concerns about the client's stools. The Bristol Stool Chart classifies faeces into seven different types. Using the Bristol Stool Chart ensures that there is consistency in reporting.

> **Task** What kinds of things do you think should be reported to your supervisor?

Bristol Stool Chart

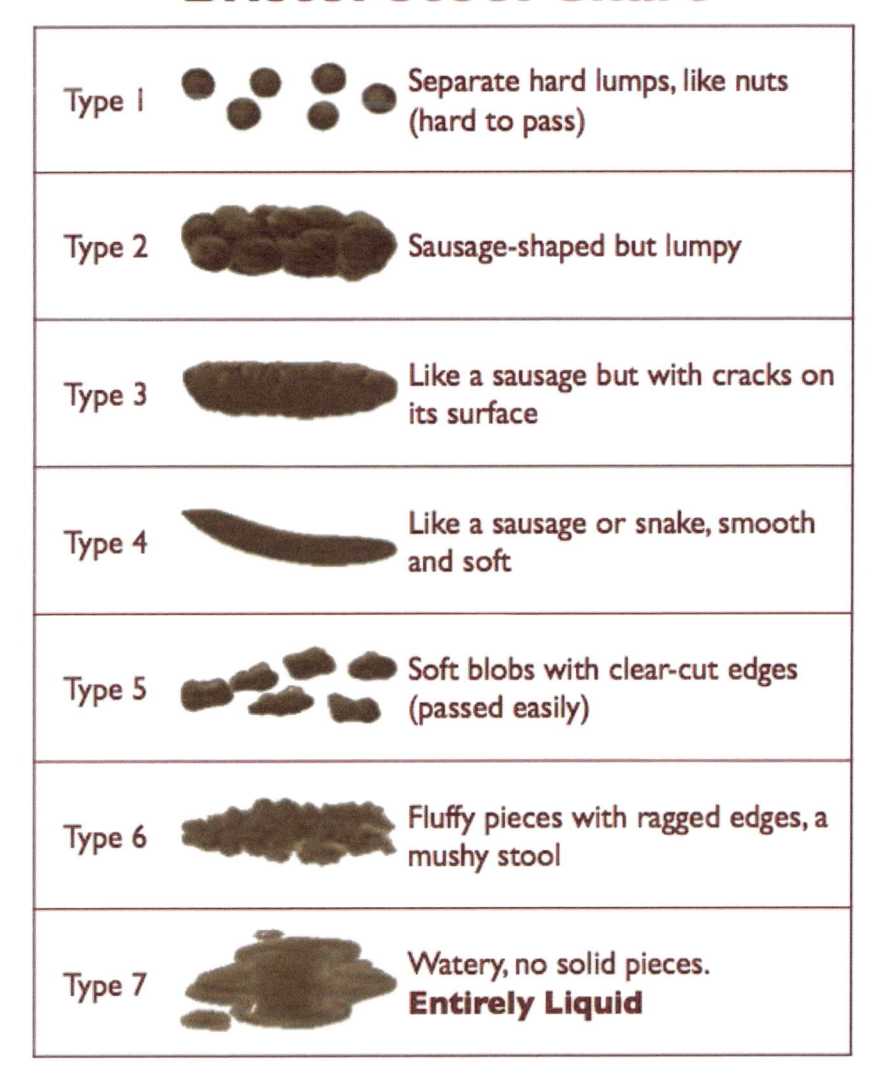

Type 1		Separate hard lumps, like nuts (hard to pass)
Type 2		Sausage-shaped but lumpy
Type 3		Like a sausage but with cracks on its surface
Type 4		Like a sausage or snake, smooth and soft
Type 5		Soft blobs with clear-cut edges (passed easily)
Type 6		Fluffy pieces with ragged edges, a mushy stool
Type 7		Watery, no solid pieces. **Entirely Liquid**

S. J. Lewis & K. W. Heaton (1997) *Stool Form Scale as a Useful Guide to Intestinal Transit Time, Scandinavian Journal of Gastroenterology*, 32:9, 920-924

Exercise:

Jack presses the nurse-call button. He is 77 years old. He can walk with a walking frame and with supervision. When you get to Jack's bedside, he tells you that he wants to go to the toilet. As Jack is walking to the toilet, he is unable to hold it any longer and is incontinent of faeces. Jack gets upset and is very embarrassed.

+ Explain what you will do to assist Jack.

Revision Questions:

1. Explain the terms 'incontinence' and 'continence'.
2. List the levels of toileting assistance that a client might require.
3. Why is maintaining a client's dignity and respect so important during toileting assistance?
4. What preparations should you make before attending to a client's toileting needs?

Key words/phrases:

commode	continence
bedpan	catheter
urinal	stoma bag
sluice room	toileting needs
incontinence	Bristol Stool Chart

HELPING WITH MOBILITY 09

Some clients will need help to move about and to mobilise. They may need help moving in the bed, getting out of the bed, standing up from their chair, and they may need help to get about.

IN THIS CHAPTER YOU WILL LEARN ABOUT:

- The different levels of help needed depending on the client's needs
- Mobility aids used to move a person or help them mobilise independently
- How to help someone to mobilise
- The importance of safety when helping someone mobilise
- The uses and advantages of manual handling aids
- Adaptions to a person's home to enable independent living
- The risk of falls and how to minimise it
- Maintaining a client's respect and dignity; treating the person as an individual; the importance of good communication; how to encourage independence
- Reporting and recording the cares given
- How to assist a wheelchair user

ASSESSING THE CLIENT'S MOBILITY NEEDS

The person you are caring for may need help with movement and walking. Each person is different, and you need to find out what help is needed.

- The client may be totally dependent on the carer for mobility.

- The person may only need supervision when walking if they are unsteady on their feet but can usually walk without help; or they may need to use a walking aid.

- The person may be able to walk unaided but need assistance to get out of bed or to go from sitting to standing.

- The person may not be able to walk and needs to use a wheelchair.

- The person may be able to move independently in the wheelchair, or you may have to push them in the wheelchair.

Plan and Prepare

To help a person with their mobility needs, you need to plan the care given. You need to know what level of care is needed and how to help them. Check the care plan and the client notes for any special instructions and talk to your supervisor or the nurse in charge. You will have information from the report or handover. Ask the client what help and how much help is needed. Then determine how many carers are needed. Will you be able to help the client on your own or will you need two carers to help the client to stand?

- **Prepare yourself:** Attend to your own hand hygiene and wear any necessary PPE. Mind your back when helping the client to mobilise. If two carers are needed, do not attempt to undertake the work on your own. Use manual handling equipment if it is needed and ensure that you have current training in manual and patient handling.

- **Prepare the client:** Introduce yourself ('Hello, my name is ...'), get consent and give explanations. Promote the client's independence by encouraging them to mobilise. Make sure that the client has suitable footwear and if necessary assist them with their footwear.

- **Prepare the environment:** Get any equipment or walking aids needed. Move furniture and any obstacles as necessary.

SAFETY

- Maintain safety when helping the client to mobilise.

- Make sure that the floor is not wet or slippery.

- Make sure that the area is free of objects and clutter that the client could trip over.

- Manual handling aids can be used to reduce the risk of back injury to the carer, making it easier to move the client.

- **Mind your back!** Helping a client out of bed or to sit up from a chair carries a risk to your back. Always follow safe manual handling guidelines and use any manual handling aids necessary. You must be trained in safe manual and patient handling and your training certificate must be in date.

Looking After Your Back

Be kind to your back: it's the only one you've got!

- Always bend from the hips and knees.

- Keep your back and neck straight.

- Keep your feet shoulder-width apart.

- Stand as close as possible to the person you're moving.

Remember – you cannot take care of someone else if you become sick or injured!

Communication

Always communicate with the client while you are helping them to mobilise. They may need reassurance – sometimes older clients have a fear of falling and this affects their self-confidence. They can feel anxious and reluctant to mobilise, but letting them know that you are with them can help. Regular walking and exercise will maintain muscle and bone strength and improve their balance. They may be afraid to walk in case they fall, but regular walks will reduce their risk of falling.

Don't rush them. Give them guidance as they are mobilising. Even when a client is standing up from a chair or sitting down on a chair, you may need to remind them of what to do. Give simple and clear instructions.

ASSISTING WITH MOBILITY

Helping a Client Transfer in the Bed

The person you are looking after may need assistance to move in bed. They may want to sit up in bed or turn in the bed. Encourage independence when helping someone to move in bed. They may be able to move themselves with clear and simple instructions.

Always ensure safety and mind your back. If two carers are needed, do not attempt to move the client on your own. Use pillows to help support the person and use any moving aids available. Remember to follow the usual steps: plan and prepare; assist the client; report and record.

There are several **manual handling aids** available to help the client to move themselves in bed.

- A bed rail can help a client to climb out of bed independently.
- Bed rails with bumpers can make the client feel safe in the bed and reduce the risk of injury. **Important:** Bed rails must be used

with caution and a risk assessment should be carried out to determine if the client is suitable for bed rails (See p. 57 for more information).

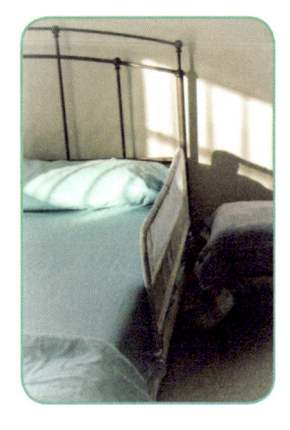

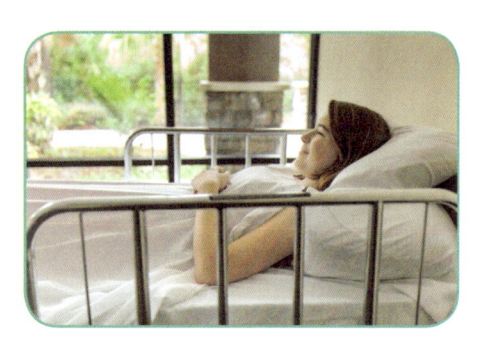

- A bed rope ladder fits around the legs of the bed and can be used by the client to pull themselves from a lying to a sitting position.

- Over-bed grab rails (sometimes called monkey poles) can be used by the client to help themselves to sit up, or to change their own position, preventing pressure sores forming.

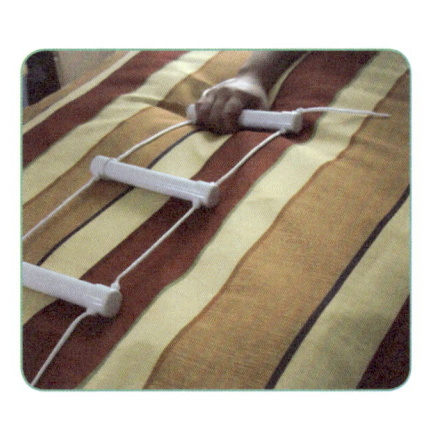

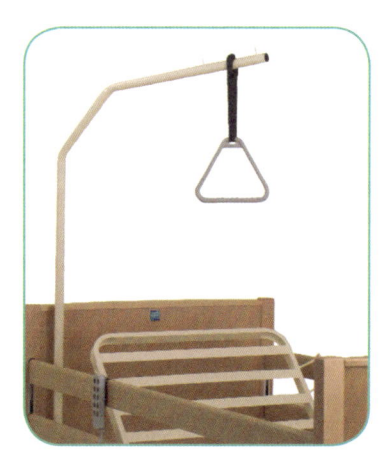

- Beds that can be lowered, have the back raised or the foot of the bed raised help to make the client more comfortable. Special alternating pressure mattresses can help reduce the risk of getting pressure sores.

- A sliding sheet is a low-friction sheet that is placed under the client in bed to help them to turn. The client wears a transfer belt around their waist to help hold them safely when transferring.

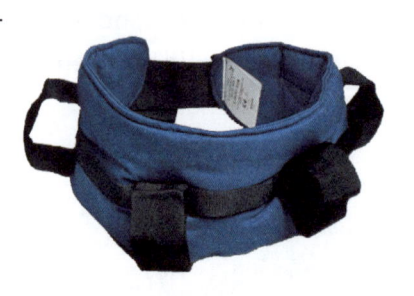

> A full-length transfer slide/board called a PAT slide is commonly used to transfer a client from bed to a trolley. A banana board is used to transfer a client from a seated position in a bed or chair to a wheelchair.

Helping a Client Transfer from Bed to Chair

How you assist a client transfer from bed to chair depends on a number of factors:

- What is the dependency level of the client?
- Is there an underlying condition that needs to be considered when transferring the client?
- Are there any attachments, such as intravenous lines or catheters?
- Are there any special medical instructions?

Plan and Prepare

- **Consult the care plan:** Talk to the supervisor/nurse in charge and consult the client.
- **Prepare yourself:** Attend to hand hygiene, wear PPE if needed, ensure you are wearing suitable clothing that allows free movement and flat non-slip shoes.

- **Prepare the client:** Introduce yourself, give clear explanations and get the consent of the client. Ensure that the client is wearing safe, non-slip footwear.

- **Prepare the environment:** Move any furniture you need to make space to safely manoeuvre. You may need to bring the chair close to the bed or move the bed if necessary. Get any equipment needed such as handling belts or mechanical aids.

Assisting the Client

- Encourage independence and give the client clear step-by-step instructions.

- Ensure the client's privacy. In some situations, it may be necessary to screen the area or ensure that the patient is adequately clothed and will not be exposed during the procedure.

- Assist the client to sit at the side of the bed with feet touching the floor.

- Remember safety. If transferring to a commode or a wheelchair, check that the brakes are on.

- **Mind your back** and don't attempt to assist a client to transfer if you feel they are at risk of falling or are unsteady. Two carers may be needed.

- If using a walking frame, bring it close to the client. Encourage them to push off the bed with one hand while placing the other hand on the walking frame.

- When the client is standing, allow them time to be confident that they have their balance.

- Don't rush the client.

- Give clear instructions on how to use the walking frame to take steps from the bed to the chair. Give instructions on turning and taking backward steps until they feel the chair at the back of their legs.

+ Instruct them on gently lowering themselves down into the chair, with one hand on the armrest of the chair, and the other hand on the walking frame.

After the Transfer

+ Place any equipment the client needs within their reach, including the nurse-call button.

+ Clean and store any equipment used.

+ Remove any PPE and attend to hand hygiene.

+ Report and document assistance given.

Helping a Client Stand Up from a Chair

When helping an individual with limited mobility stand up or transfer from one location to another, your own personal safety is just as important as theirs. Poor transfer techniques can lead to back injuries and an increased risk of accidents, such as falls, which can injure both the client and the carer.

Plan and Prepare

+ **Check the client's care plan:** Consult with the supervisor/nurse in charge, and the client. Check how many carers are needed.

+ **Prepare yourself:** Hand hygiene, use of PPE, appropriate clothing and footwear.

+ **Prepare the client:** Introduce yourself, give clear, step-by-step explanations and get consent. Make sure the client is wearing suitable non-slip footwear.

- **Prepare the environment:** Move furniture as necessary to allow room to manoeuvre, make sure there are no obstructions, and get any equipment needed, such as a handling belt.

Assisting the Client

- Advise the client that they will need to push up from the chair arms and keep their head up. Follow a simple prompting regime, for example, 'Ready, steady, stand', to ensure co-ordination.

- Ensure the client's privacy. In some situations it may be necessary to screen the area. Make sure that the patient is adequately clothed and is not going to be exposed during the procedure.

- Ensure that the chair is secure and not going to move. If the chair has wheels, check that the brakes are on.

- If the client is going to use a walking frame, position it close to them.

- Ask the client to position themselves to prepare them for standing. Ask them to move forward in the chair and then to wriggle or shuffle to the front of the chair, bringing their shoulders forward and not leaning backwards.

- Make sure that the client's feet are flat on the floor, slightly apart, usually hip width, and with one foot slightly in front of the other.

- Ask the client not to look down at the floor when standing but to lift their head up.

- Ask the client to position their hands on the chair arms.

- When the client is ready, say 'Ready, steady, stand', advising them to stand by pushing up from the chair arms.

- Check that the client is steady.

Mechanical Aids

A standing hoist is used to assist a client from a sitting to a standing position. Hoists can be attached to the ceiling, or mobile hoists are moved from client to client. The client lies in a sling and the hoist is used to raise them up and move them. It is very important that the carer is trained in using the hoist and knows how to use it correctly.

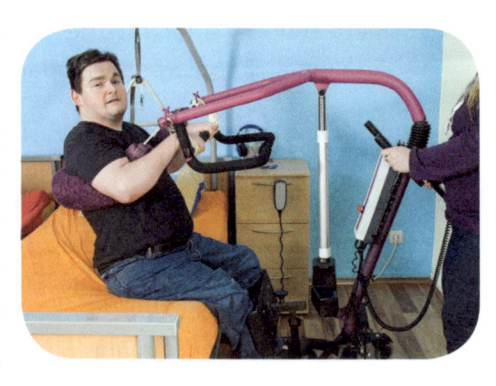

Helping a Client to Move About

Mobility aids are devices designed to help people with problems moving around and to give them greater freedom and independence. These aids can also reduce pain and increase confidence and self-esteem. The type of mobility aid required will depend on the client's issues or needs.

Walking Sticks

Walking sticks are useful for people who may be a little unsteady on their feet from time to time or at risk of falling. They support the body's weight and help transmit the load from the legs to the upper body, but they can place greater pressure on the hands and wrists.

Types of walking sticks:

- **White sticks** are used by people who are visually impaired. They are longer and thinner than traditional walking sticks to allow the user to detect objects in their path. They also inform other people that the user is blind or visually impaired.

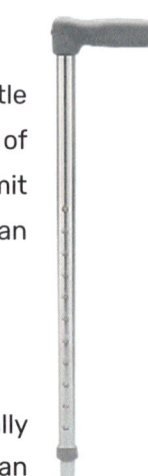

+ **Quad walking sticks** have four feet at the end of the cane, providing a wider base and greater stability for the client.

+ **Walkers or Zimmer frames** have a metal framework with four legs and provide stability and support to the user. Basic walkers have a three-sided frame that surrounds the front of the user. The frame is lifted and placed further in front of them, and then they step forward to meet it. Some walkers have wheels or glides on the base of the legs, allowing the user to slide the walker rather than lift it. This is more suitable for people with limited arm strength.

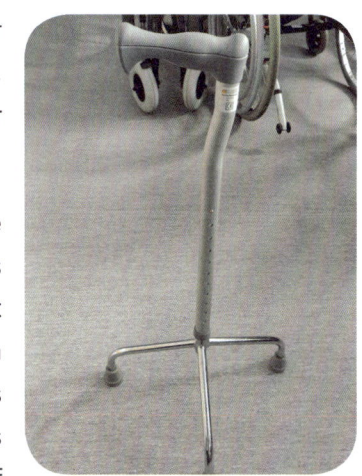

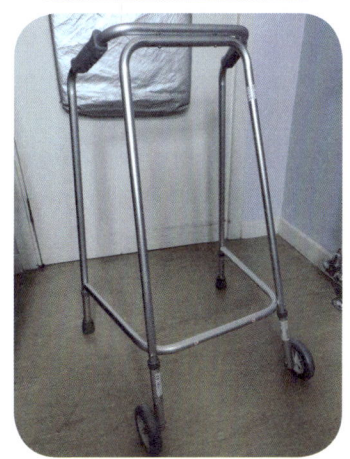

Wheelchairs

Wheelchairs are used by people who should not or cannot put weight on their lower limbs or who are unable to walk. A client who uses a wheelchair may need very little assistance or may need full assistance. Assess the wheelchair user individually to determine how much assistance is needed.

Getting into the Wheelchair

The client may be able to transfer into their wheelchair without assistance. They may need a small amount of assistance, such as positioning the wheelchair for them and making sure that the wheelchair brakes are on. The client may need to use a transfer board (banana board) to transfer from a seated position in the bed or a chair to a wheelchair. Position the wheelchair close to the client.

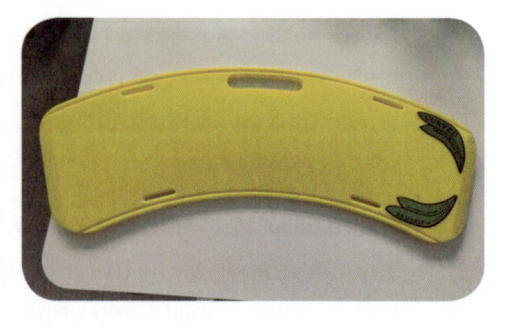

Remove the armrest of the wheelchair to make it easier for the client to transfer across, making sure that the brakes are on. The footplates should be folded up and the footrests turned back. This gives room for the client to transfer and prevents them banging their legs against the footrest. Assist the client as necessary.

When the client has safely transferred to the wheelchair, replace the armrest, bring the footrests forward and turn down the footplates. Assist the client to place their feet on the footrests.

When the client is in the wheelchair, they may be able to independently mobilise, or they may need the carer to push the wheelchair.

> There are different types of wheelchair. Manual wheelchairs may need to be pushed by a carer, or the client may be able to move themselves by propelling the wheels. These wheelchairs can be folded up when not in use. Electric wheelchairs come in different sizes and designs.

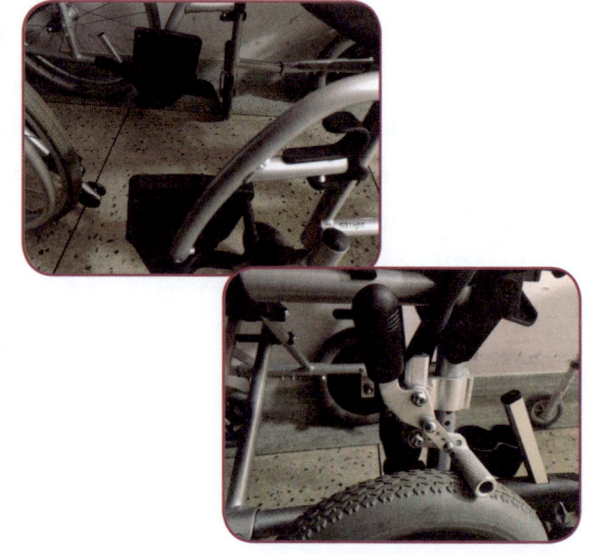

PRACTICAL TIPS FOR ASSISTING WITH MOBILITY

When helping a person to mobilise it is important to encourage independence. Using mobility aids can help a client to mobilise safely, but they are of little use unless the client can reach them. If they have to be stored safely when not in use, make sure that the client has access to a nurse-call button to get the attention of a carer when they need to mobilise.

Good muscle strength and balance are important when mobilising; for this the clients may need to attend physiotherapy sessions. Exercise and activity sessions should be encouraged to build up strong muscles and balance.

Maintain the client's respect and dignity when helping them to mobilise. Good communication is important, and instructions should be given clearly and simply. Don't rush the client and always remain calm.

Adaptations in the Home

People who need care can live in their own home if the home is adapted to their needs. These adaptations can include ramps, stairlifts, grab rails, wide doors for wheelchair access, adapted bathrooms and toilets.

> **Task** Research the adaptations that can be made to the house of a client using a wheelchair to enable them to live to their fullest potential.

Exercise:

Peggy is 67 and has rheumatoid arthritis. She has difficulty mobilising and finds the activities for day-to-day living difficult. She lives alone. She wants to be as independent as possible.

+ Suggest ways in which Peggy can continue to live independently with the use of care aids.

MANUAL HANDLING REGULATIONS

Important Note!

The Safety, Health and Welfare at Work (General Application) Regulations 2007, Chapter 4 of Part 2 (S.I. No.299 of 2007), also known as the Manual Handling of Loads Regulation, outline the requirements that must be fulfilled in relation to manual handling. Manual handling of loads is defined in the regulation and includes any lifting, putting down, pushing, pulling, carrying or moving of a load which, by reason of its characteristics or unfavourable ergonomic conditions, involves risk, particularly of back injury, to employees.

The basic principle is that where manual handling of loads involving a risk of injury (particularly to the back) is present, the employer must take measures to avoid or reduce the risk of injury.

Three key requirements in this regulation are:

1. Avoiding manual handling activities that involve a risk of injury.

2. Risk assessment of manual handling tasks that cannot be avoided.

3. Reduction of the risk from manual handling activities.

The HSE operates a 'Minimal Handling Policy', which states that in the case of people handling, an assessment will include the manual handling needs of the client and the safest way of undertaking these tasks. This is achieved through good planning, consultation and the systematic management of risks by providing: a safe working environment; safe systems of work; adequate information, instruction, training and supervision; and suitable aids and equipment. The principles of ergonomics will be applied in the design and refurbishment of workplaces and when purchasing equipment and furniture (HSA 2011; HSE 2018a).

Task What manual handling aids are used in your workplace? Describe how they are used.

When using mobility aids, follow the instructions carefully and assess the client's suitability for use of the aid.

FALLS RISKS

Some clients you are caring for may be at risk of falling, e.g. an elderly resident in a nursing home. The client will be assessed using a **Falls Risk Assessment Chart** (see Appendix 7) to see if they are classed as being at risk of falling. Falls can lead to injuries, such as fractured bones, as well as fear and lack of confidence.

Older people are particularly at risk of falling, due to:

- **Lack of physical activity:** Lack of regular exercise can result in decreased strength, muscle tone, flexibility and bone strength.

- **Impaired vision:** Age-related vision diseases can increase the risk of a person falling. Cataracts and glaucoma can alter an older person's depth perception and peripheral vision.
- **Medications:** All medicines have potential side effects, and some side effects can increase the risk of falling.

Other situations that can lead to falls include:

- Poor lighting. Make sure all areas are well lit, including hallways, entrances and exits. A touch light beside the bed to make it easy to turn the light on and off is a good idea.
- Lack of handrails. Clients should use handrails in the bathroom to help keep their balance.
- Loose flooring – rugs or carpets that are not properly secured.
- Wet floors.
- Storage areas, e.g. cupboards that a client has to stretch to reach.
- The client rushing to get to the toilet during the day or at night.
- Chairs with wheels.
- Chairs without armrests.
- Walking in bare feet, open-back shoes or loose slippers (HSE 'Preventing Falls' leaflet).

Preventing Falls in Healthcare: Think ACE!

The HSE advocates investigating a client's falls history either at home or in care, as this is the strongest predictor of future falling. The ACE plan – **A**ssess, **C**are and **E**valuate – involves assessing the client on admission or at initial consultation; discussing their falls history;

devising a care plan that includes their personal and environmental factors; and evaluating the client's falls risk weekly, or if their criteria changes or if they fall (HSE 2012b).

AFTER HELPING THE CLIENT

- Safely remove and discard any PPE and attend to your own hand hygiene.

- Record and report: If you have any concerns about the client's mobility or see a change – either improvement or deterioration – report it to the nurse in charge or your supervisor.

- Complete the client's care plans.

> **Exercise:**
>
> Josie is 87 years old and living at home. She has a home help who visits her twice a day. She has recently had several falls. Although she was not badly hurt, Josie has lost confidence and has a fear of falling. She wants to remain living at home. She lives in a two-storey house with narrow stairs. She sleeps upstairs, and her bathroom is upstairs. She does not have a downstairs bathroom. Over the years she has accumulated a good deal of furniture and has loose rugs and mats on the floor.
>
> You are asked to perform a risk assessment of Josie's home to determine the risks of Josie falling.
>
> - Suggest to Josie ways in which she can prevent any further falls and continue living safely in her own home.

> **Revision Questions:**
>
> 1. Why is communication important when assisting a client with mobility?
> 2. List the levels of mobility that a client might have.
> 3. What preparations do you undertake before you assist a client with mobility?
> 4. Why are manual handling guidelines so important?
> 5. List four dangers in the home or room that can cause an elderly person to fall.

> **Key words/phrases:**
>
> mobility
>
> falls risk assessment
>
> mobility aids

PREVENTING PRESSURE SORES 10

Some people you will care for may have difficulty moving or walking and some may be bedridden. These people may be at risk of getting pressure sores or bedsores, which affect areas of the skin and underlying tissue. They are caused when the affected area of skin is placed under too much pressure. Pressure sores can range in severity from patches of discoloured skin to open wounds that expose the underlying bone or muscle. They are slow to heal and can cause much discomfort and pain. The goal for carers is to prevent clients developing a pressure sore.

IN THIS CHAPTER YOU WILL LEARN ABOUT:

- What a pressure sore is
- Stages of pressure sores
- Common sites for pressure sores
- Causes of pressure sores and risk factors
- How to prevent pressure sores

WHAT IS A PRESSURE SORE?

Pressure sores, or pressure ulcers, are sometimes called bedsores because those most likely to develop them are bedridden or restricted to bed and unable to move themselves or adjust their position.

They develop when a large amount of pressure is applied to an area of skin over a short period of time, or when less force is applied but over a longer period.

If you lie in the same position, without moving, the skin becomes compressed. This compression or extra pressure disrupts the flow of blood through the skin. Without a blood supply, the affected area of skin becomes starved of oxygen and nutrients and becomes damaged. It begins to break down, leading to the formation of a pressure sore.

We see this damage first as a change in the colour of the skin. If the pressure continues, the skin will break down, and the muscles under the skin may also become damaged. In the worst cases the damage can extend all the way down to the bone.

> **Red is a warning.** Red skin is usually your first sign of a pressure sore.

Healthy people do not get pressure sores because they are continuously and subconsciously adjusting their posture and position so that no part of their body is subjected to excessive pressure.

However, people with health conditions that make it difficult for them to move their body often develop pressure sores. In addition, conditions that can affect the flow of blood through the body, such as type 2 diabetes, can make a person more vulnerable to pressure sores.

Remember: a pressure sore is caused by prolonged pressure when the client has been lying or sitting in the same position for too long (HSE website, 'Bed Sores').

HOW TO ASSESS A PRESSURE SORE

The European Pressure Ulcer Advisory Panel (EPUAP) assesses pressure sores according to their depth.

CHAPTER 10: PREFENTING PRESSURE SORES

- Stage 1: Skin redness that doesn't turn white under pressure.

- Stage 2: A scrape or blister that results from loss of the outer skin layers.

- Stage 3: A shallow crater from loss of the dermis and subcutaneous layers of skin.

- Stage 4: Tissue necrosis (death of tissues) and full-thickness skin loss, often with tunnelling sinus tracts.

Category / Stage I

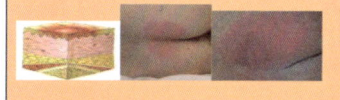

Category/ Stage I: Intact skin with non – blanchable redness of a localised area usually over a bony prominence. Discolouration of the skin, warmth, odema, hardness or pain may also be present. Darkly pigmented skin may not have visible blanching. The area may be painful, firm, soft, warmer or cooler as compared to adjacent skin. (EPUAP 2009).

Category/Stage II

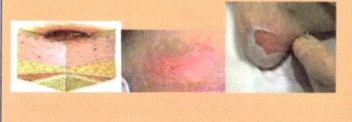

Category / Stage II: Partial thickness skin loss of dermis presenting as a shallow ulcer with a red pink wound bed, without slough. May present as an intact or open/ ruptured serum filled blister filled with serous or sero- sanginous fluid. Presents as a shiny or dry shallow ulcer without slough or bruising. (EPUAP 2009).

Category/Stage III

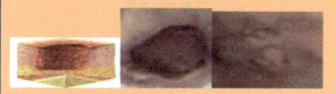

Category / Stage III: Full thickness skin loss. Subcutaneous fat may be visible but bone, tendon or muscles are not exposed. Slough may be present but does not obscure the depth of tissue loss. The stage may include undermining or tunnelling (EPUAP 2009).

Category/Stage IV

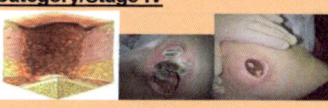

Category / Stage IV: Full thickness tissue loss with exposed bone, tendon or muscle. Slough or eschar may be present. This stage often includes undermining and tunnelling. Exposed bone / muscle

Suspected deep pressure and shear induced tissue damage, depth unknown

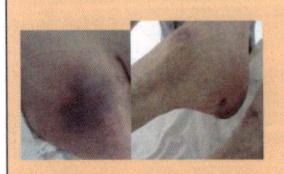

In individuals with non-blanchable redness and purple/maroon discoloration of intact skin combined with a history of prolonged, unrelieved pressure/shear, this skin change may be an indication of emerging, more severe pressure ulceration i.e. an emerging **Category/Stage III or IV Pressure Ulcer**. Clear recording of the exact nature of the visible skin changes, including recording of the risk that these changes may be an indication of emerging more severe pressure ulceration, should be documented in the patients' health record. These observations should be recorded in tandem with information pertaining to the patient history of prolonged, unrelieved pressure/shear.

It is estimated that it could take **3-10 days** from the initial insult causing the damage, to become a **Category/Stage III or IV Pressure Ulcer** (Black et al, 2015).

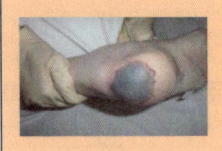

Stable eschar (dry adherent, intact without erythema or fluctuance) on the heel serves as the body's biological cover and should not be removed. It should be documented as at least Category / Stage III until proven otherwise.

Source: Pressure Ulcers, A Practical Guide, HSE (2018)

You can get a pressure sore in any part of the body where there are bony prominences.

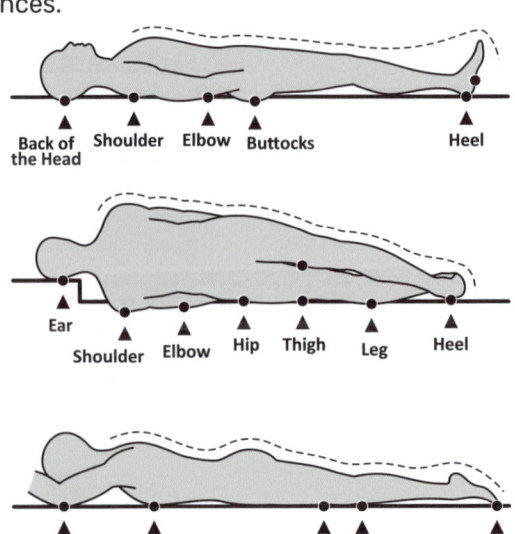

Back of the Head, Shoulder, Elbow, Buttocks, Heel

Ear, Shoulder, Elbow, Hip, Thigh, Leg, Heel

Elbow, Rib Cage, Thigh, Knees, Toes

CARING FOR A PERSON AT RISK OF GETTING A PRESSURE SORE

It can be difficult to treat a pressure sore; they cause a great deal of discomfort to the client; and they can be costly to treat. The aim of carers is to prevent a pressure sore forming.

Assess the Risk

How likely is it that the person you are looking after will get a pressure sore? There are risk factors that make some individuals more likely to get a pressure sore. Risk assessment charts, such as the **Waterlow Chart** (see Appendix 3), can be used to assess the client's risk. The chart needs to be completed when you first assess the client, and on a regular basis after this.

The risk factors are: extremes of age (very young and very old), thinning skin, chronic diseases, reduced mobility, poor nutrition/weight loss or obesity, dehydration, incontinence, sensory impairment, acute illness, level of consciousness, vascular disease and previous history of pressure damage.

Three questions to ask are:

- Can the person move themselves?
- Are they incontinent?
- Are they eating and drinking?

If your client has difficulty moving, is incontinent and not eating and drinking sufficiently, they are at risk of getting a pressure sore, and you must take steps to prevent this happening.

Assess the Skin

Assess the skin regularly and document what you see. Check the most vulnerable areas (sacrum, buttocks, heels, hips). The signs to look for are: purplish/bluish patches on dark-skinned people and red patches on light-skinned people, swelling, blisters, shiny areas, dry patches, cracks, calluses, wrinkles. Feel for hard areas, warm areas and swelling.

Reducing the Risk of a Pressure Sore

Frequent Change of Position

Encourage the client to change their position on their own and to mobilise. If they are unable to move themselves, the carer must change their position frequently. In practice, dependent clients must have their position changed every two hours. This needs to be documented, for example on a **turns chart** (see Appendix 4), which records what position the client is in and when their position was changed (HSE, 'Prevention of Pressure Ulcers').

The 30° tilt is a position recommended for clients who need to have their position changed frequently. It avoids pressure being placed over bony prominences, and it is comfortable for the client (HSE 2018b).

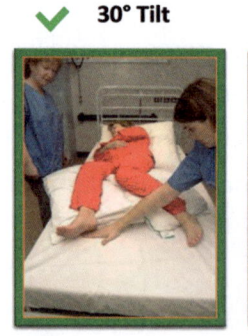

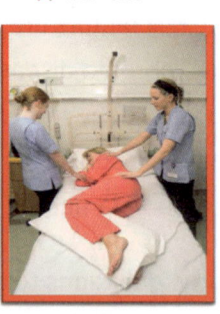

✓ 30° Tilt   ✗ 90° Tilt

(Moore et al., 2011)

Limit chair sitting to two hours. This is because sitting in a chair can put the client at high risk of getting a pressure sore if they are unable to move themselves. When you are sitting down for two hours or more you don't develop a pressure sore because you are constantly fidgeting, even if you don't realise it. Clients at risk of getting a pressure sores are not able to make these little movements.

Clients who use wheelchairs may need to have their position changed as frequently as every fifteen or thirty minutes.

Skin Care

Keep the skin clean and dry and take particular care of the skin of incontinent clients. Keep the skin moisturised and use barrier creams.

Nutrition and Hydration

Encourage good nutrition and fluid intake. Make sure that the client is eating and drinking. If necessary, the client may be referred to a dietitian.

Careful Handling

Handle the client carefully and maintain good manual handling practice. This is to avoid friction or rubbing of the skin against the bedclothes.

Pressure-relieving Aids

At-risk clients should use a special air mattress called an alternating pressure mattress, which changes the pressure under the client's body by inflating or deflating the air in the bed. However, the client's position still needs to be changed regularly.

Educate the Client and their Family

Empower the client by letting them know the importance of changing their position. Let them know what they can do for themselves and help them recognise the early signs of a pressure sore. Remember, always give explanations to the client and get their consent before delivering any cares. Promote independence by encouraging the client to move themselves. Pressure sores often occur on the client's buttocks and sacral area, so they may feel embarrassed by this; remember, always respect the dignity of the client when assessing the skin.

RECORD AND REPORT

Keep records of the steps taken to prevent pressure sores and of the assessment of the skin. Any changes to the skin or any increased risk must be reported to the nurse in charge or your supervisor. Assessment of the client's risk is recorded by the nurse on a pressure sore risk assessment tool, such as the Waterlow Chart (see Appendix 2). When the client's position is changed, this should be recorded on a turns chart (see Appendix 4).

Exercise:

Jack is 97 years old. He is tall and underweight. He has had a stroke, which has left him unable to move independently or change his own position. He needs assistance with eating and drinking. He is incontinent of faeces and urine and wears incontinence pads.

- Explain why Jack is at risk of getting a pressure sore.
- Discuss four ways in which you could help prevent Jack getting a pressure sore.

Revision Questions:

1. What are the risk factors for developing pressure sores?
2. What are the key signs of pressure sores developing?
3. List the stages of the development of pressure sores.
4. How are pressures sores treated?
5. How are pressure sores prevented?

Key words/phrases:

pressure sores/ulcers	shallow craters
bedridden	tissue necrosis
skin redness	Waterlow Chart
blisters	alternating pressure mattress

CLEANLINESS AND PREVENTING THE SPREAD OF INFECTION

11

The carer has a very important role in maintaining a clean and safe environment. If the workplace and the equipment are not cleaned thoroughly it can lead to the spread of infections and illness. The people you are caring for are often at high risk of getting infections. If they are already weakened, due to old age or illness, getting an infection can be very serious. The carer must follow the workplace policy and procedures with regard to cleanliness and hygiene. Strict adherence to good cleanliness can minimise the risk of infections spreading.

IN THIS CHAPTER YOU WILL LEARN ABOUT:

- The importance of cleaning and safely storing care equipment and the steps to follow in correct cleaning and storage
- Maintaining cleanliness in the care environment
- The safe management of linen and handling dirty laundry
- The safe management of waste

CLEANING CARE EQUIPMENT AND THE ENVIRONMENT

Cleaning involves the removal of dirt from the equipment used by the client and from the environment.

> Revise Chapter 5 Hygiene.

Care Equipment

All care equipment must be stored clean and dry following use. Equipment should also be checked for cleanliness before it is used. It should be checked and cleaned regularly. Care equipment should be free from blood or other bodily fluids, dirt, dust or rust. Care equipment needs to be cleaned daily and after use. It should also be cleaned after a spillage or contamination.

The carer will be responsible for safe cleanliness and storage of:

- Bowls for washing: After use, clean, dry thoroughly and store upside down in the client's room.
- Bedpans, urinals and buckets from commodes: Rinse after use and place in the bedpan washer. Store safely in the sluice room.
- Commodes: Clean after each use; thoroughly clean on a regular basis according to workplace policy.

When performing procedures for the management of care equipment:

- Use personal protective equipment (PPE).
- Remember hand hygiene.
- Follow local procedure in relation to cleaning agent, receptacle and products to be used.
- Follow the local policy for cleaning equipment.

Care Environment

The term 'environment' refers to any general horizontal surfaces in the client's environment and any frequently touched surfaces in the environment, such as:

- beds and trolleys
- chairs and other furniture in the environment
- bedside items such as lockers and tables, bedside telephones and televisions
- toilets and commodes
- sinks, basins, baths and showers and the items surrounding them
- hand hygiene solution containers
- floors
- doors, door handles
- paintwork and surroundings
- curtains/screens, window blinds
- light fittings and light switches
- kitchen areas.

> Remember! Proper dress code, hand hygiene practices and appropriate use of PPE is essential in reducing the spread of infections.

General guidelines for the environment include:

- **Smooth surfaces:** All client environments are at risk of contamination, and must be controlled. Environmental surfaces must be smooth without any cracks or breaks. Any cracks or roughness can harbour germs.

- **Tidy and clutter-free:** There should be ample storage space for the client's belongings and for all stored equipment. Clutter and mess can lead to slips and trips, which are one of the most common causes of accidents in the workplace.

- **Good working order:** The equipment used in a care environment must be in good working order and comply with safety regulations. The equipment should be easy to clean and any equipment or furnishings that are damaged or broken should be removed.

- **Reporting:** Report any damaged equipment to your supervisor. Many workplaces have a maintenance worker who regularly sees to repairs. There is likely to be a reporting system to alert the maintenance worker to any repairs (www.hsa.ie).

SAFE MANAGEMENT OF LINEN

In the care setting the carer will have to deal with linen, such as bedclothes. Bed-making is a part of the carer's work day. It's important that dirty bedclothes and laundry are dealt with correctly to minimise the spread of infections. Soiled laundry in care settings can harbour large numbers of potentially disease-carrying germs.

The following HSE guidelines give clear instructions on how to deal with clean and dirty linen.

- Perform hand hygiene before handling clean linen.

- Handle used linen carefully to avoid contaminating the environment. For example, used laundry should not be shaken or placed on the floor or any clean surfaces.

- Wear PPE when you anticipate being in contact with laundry and linen soiled with blood or bodily fluids, secretions and excretions (except sweat).

- Do not manually sluice soiled laundry.

- Items soiled with blood or body fluids should be placed in red/orange alginate stitched bags or water-soluble bags.

> The red/orange alginate water-soluble bag signifies that the laundry is foul/infected.

- Ensure that laundry is free from sharps waste and foreign objects such as incontinence wear.

- All dirty linen must be placed carefully and directly into the appropriate laundry bag on removal from the bed or patient. Bring the laundry skip to the bedside and place dirty linen into the appropriate bag.

- Perform hand hygiene after handling used linen.

Linen can be classified into three categories. The HSE guidelines explain how to deal with each category.

1. Clean/unused linen:

    - Any linen that has not been used since it was last laundered.

    - All clean linen must be stored off the floor in a clean, closed cupboard and must be segregated from dirty/used linen. It must not be stored in the sluice or bathroom. Linen cupboard doors must be kept closed to prevent airborne contamination.

2. Foul/infected linen:

    - Any used linen that is soiled with blood or any other body fluid.

    - All linen used by a patient with a known infection (soiled or not).

    - All dirty/infected linen must be placed in a red/orange soluble alginate bag which is secured by the neck using an alginate tie or swan neck tie.

- Foul/infected linen should be transported to the laundry in a red laundry bag.

- The soluble bag must be placed directly into the washing machine to minimise contact and prevent transmission of infection to laundry staff or contamination of the environment. If at any time an item of laundry is so heavily contaminated with blood or other body fluids that it is deemed unsalvageable, it should be risk-assessed and placed in either a risk waste or non-risk waste bag for disposal.

3. Dirty/used linen:

    - All used linen other than that listed above – this includes coloured items and scrubs and theatre linen.

    - Body linen, including underclothing, day and night wear, woollen articles and all coloured dirty used linen must be segregated from white linen as part of the laundry process, and should be placed in **blue laundry bags**.

    - Dirty used theatre linen, usually green, should be placed in a **water-soluble or alginate bag**. The secured bag should be placed into a **green laundry bag** for transportation to the laundry.

    - All other used dirty linen that falls within this category must be placed into a plain clear plastic bag identifying it as dirty/used linen and transported to the laundry in a **white laundry bag** (HSE 2006).

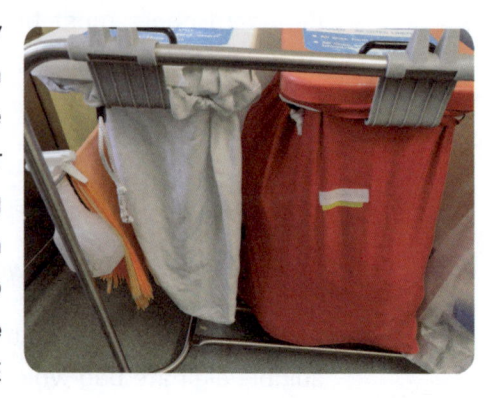

SAFE WASTE MANAGEMENT

The carer must dispose of waste in a safe manner to prevent the spread of infection.

- Waste should be disposed of as close to the point of use as possible, immediately after use.

- Use hands-free/pedal-operated lids, hard-bodied and strong, containing appropriate waste bags, so that hands do not become contaminated during waste disposal, e.g. by having to touch the lid to open it.

- Yellow bin-bags indicate hazardous healthcare waste for treatment/incineration and disposal.

- Examples of infectious waste include:
  - blood and items visibly soiled from blood
  - contaminated waste from patients with infectious diseases
  - incontinence wear/nappies from patients with known or suspected enteric pathogens
  - items contaminated with body fluids other than faeces, urine or breast milk.

- Sharps: any object which has been used in the diagnosis, treatment or prevention of disease that is likely to cause a puncture wound or cut to the skin. These must be placed in puncture-resistant sharps containers/boxes for sharps.

- Never dispose of waste in an already full receptacle.

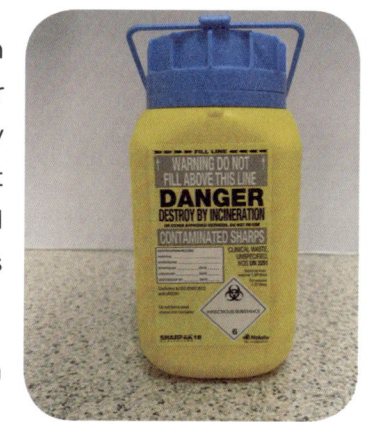

- Bags should be no more than three-quarters full. Sharps bins should be no more than three-quarters full or past the manufacturer's fill line.

Guidelines for Safe Waste Disposal

- Always wear PPE.
- Never touch the waste receptacle itself and never over-fill waste receptacles.
- Seal all bags/containers appropriately before disposal.
- Perform hand hygiene following any waste handling/disposal.
- Manage spillages in line with local policy.

Task

You are asked to assist a client with their hygiene needs. The client has been incontinent of urine and faeces and the bedlinen is soiled. The client has a wound to their lower leg and this has been bleeding.

Explain how you will attend to cleanliness and hygiene while assisting the client to wash.

Revision Questions:

1. What is the correct procedure for disposing of sharps?
2. What are the three categories of linen? How would you safely handle and deal with each category?
3. How would you prepare yourself before cleaning equipment or removing dirty linen?
4. Why is it important to be aware of and follow HSE guidelines on safe waste management?

CHAPTER 11: CLEANLINESS

Key words/phrases:

care environment

treatment rooms

sluice rooms

dirty linen

alginate bags

contaminated linen

foul/infected linen

disposal of sharps

safe waste management

SOCIAL ACTIVITIES

12

Most of us enjoy social events. We enjoy meeting and chatting to people, going for a coffee and cake or going to the cinema. We have hobbies and interests and we join clubs and societies. We play sport and we may like to be active. We do these things because they are fun, and they help to complete our lives. Even when we are busy we usually manage to squeeze in social activities. The people we are caring for also have social needs as well as physical needs. However, they sometimes need assistance to partake in social events. It is important that we help and facilitate our clients to participate in social activities. It adds an important dimension to their lives and enriches and enhances the quality of their lives.

IN THIS CHAPTER YOU WILL LEARN ABOUT:

- The benefits of socialising/engaging in activities
- Barriers to engaging in activities
- Involving clients in social events
- Gaining consent
- Encouraging involvement and independence
- Planning and preparation
- Safety
- Ideas for activities
- Cultural considerations

Regardless of a person's age, socialisation is important as it can give a sense of belonging and is part of leading a fulfilled life.

Socialisation is important for elderly people. A research study (Barbour, Clark, Jones, Veitch, 2010) showed that elderly individuals who had active social lives were happier, healthier and more likely to live longer than those who did not have an active social life. Loneliness can impair an elderly person's life, while socialising can enrich it.

THE BENEFITS OF SOCIALISING/ENGAGING IN ACTIVITIES

Socialising provides opportunities to develop new friendships, to reduce stress, to keep anxiety and depression at bay, and to help people feel useful and needed. It also stimulates the mind through conversation, singing, playing cards or bingo or any number of other activities. Socialising for elderly people is key to a healthy mind – if they are isolated, depression can set in quickly – and it improves the general quality of life.

Physical Benefits

- Socially active clients deal with stress better, which can help improve cardiovascular health and the immune system.
- A high level of socialisation in older people helps increase longevity.
- Greater fitness: clients with diverse social supports and interests benefit from exercise through their range of activities, which leads to a host of physical, mental and cognitive benefits.
- Muscle strength, fitness and mobility are retained or improved.
- Weight gain is less likely.

- Risk of falls and fractures is reduced.
- Potential for blood clots and circulation problems is reduced.
- Balance, posture and co-ordination are improved.
- Appetite and digestion improve.
- Concentration and memory improve.
- The immune system becomes more efficient.

Psychological Benefits

- Social contact, self-expression and a sense of purpose and belonging are maintained or regained.
- Through consistent socialising the likelihood of experiencing depression caused by isolation and loneliness is reduced.
- Socialising reduces anxiety levels.
- Socialising helps maintain and improve self-esteem and sense of worth.
- Cognitive benefits: positive social interactions on a consistent basis help keep clients stimulated, mentally sharp and intellectually engaged.
- Mood is lifted and alertness increased.
- Tension is eased, and it becomes easier to relax.
- Choice, control and dignity are gained.
- Sense of well-being improves.

Negative Effects of Not Socialising

Lack of involvement in activities can lead to muscles and bones weakening and joints stiffening. Urinary infections become more common, which can lead to incontinence. It can also lead to blood pressure increases, and a risk of developing pressure sores, breathing difficulties and chest infections. Sleep patterns can also be affected, and clients may feel less alert and have difficulty concentrating. Loss of confidence and skills will undoubtedly develop, which can then lead to confusion and disorientation. Clients may feel bored and become short-tempered (Troyer 2016).

BARRIERS TO ENGAGING IN ACTIVITIES

It can sometimes be difficult for your clients to socialise or engage in activities. Here are some of the most common reasons why elderly clients do not socialise or engage in activities:

- Physical ailments or injuries
- Loss of a spouse or other loved one
- Isolation and/or mobility problems
- Real or perceived cognitive decline
- Less availability of family members to assist with social activities
- Lack of confidence in their ability to integrate
- Negative stereotypes of old age, such as 'I can't do that at my age …'

Some of these barriers are more challenging than others, but it is important that carers and family members work towards overcoming them.

CLIENT'S CONSENT

The client's consent is very important before participation in activities. Find out their individual needs and interests by having a one-to-one assessment. Never make assumptions that the person you are caring for will want to participate in the activity you have planned; for example, you may assume that older people enjoy bingo, but some older people don't. Even if they're not interested in bingo, they might still enjoy the social interaction around the event.

Discuss the following with your client:

- Each activity and what it entails
- Their likes, dislikes, interests; who and what is important to them
- The everyday skills and activities that they can and cannot do and what they might like to practise
- Their culture and previous lifestyle
- Their spiritual needs and how these can best be met
- Which activities and roles they would like to keep up
- Ways of keeping them mentally stimulated and physically active.

It is important that you engage at this level with the client in order to establish what they can do, what they would like to do or could potentially try in order to gain the many benefits from engaging in activities.

ENCOURAGING INVOLVEMENT IN ACTIVITIES

If you feel that your client would benefit from taking part in an activity that they do not want to do, you may be able to give them gentle encouragement to participate – but do not force the issue.

You could also give them some minor responsibilities in relation to some activities to encourage them to participate and to build their self-confidence and independence.

If they have been recently bereaved of their life partner and are reluctant to socialise, consider attending the event with them initially or by introducing them to a client who is in a similar position but who still enjoys socialising. They may be able to help each other through this difficult stage of trying to establish new routines and finding one's new identity without a partner.

Here are some tips to encourage – but not force – a client to partake in activities:

- Use humour, kindness and encouragement. Take a rational approach, such as discussing the benefits of joining in.

- Be enthusiastic and positive, but try not to sound patronising.

- Know that a gentle, caring and nurturing approach can instil confidence and promote action.

- Give responsibility by allowing clients to make a choice for themselves from a selection of activities.

If a client refuses to participate in an activity or an outing, they should never be forced or coerced. However, a different approach or ideas for solutions may be required.

TYPES OF ACTIVITY

You can introduce a myriad of activities to find ones that are appealing, interesting and enjoyable for your client. We all have different preferences, talents and interests, so it is important to remember the individuality of each client. Once you have identified your client's needs, abilities and interests, you can select the appropriate activities.

- **Cognitive activities** involve memory, concentration, sequencing, reminiscence and orientation and include activities such as word games (crosswords, 'Hangman', word chains), quizzes, board games, debates or discussions, memory games, jigsaw puzzles, writing a newsletter/magazine, being part of a residents' committee, using computers.

- **Communication** can involve discussions, storytelling, reminiscence, reading and writing, social activities, emailing, using Skype and social networks.

- **Creative activities** can include art workshops and craft activities.

- **Music activities** can involve reminiscence, theme-based quizzes, games to music, music appreciation, making or playing music, singing.

- **Physical activities** involve movement, ranging from moving to music to very active dancing, and can also include ball games, exercise (both seated and standing), falls prevention programmes, Tai Chi, Wii games, encouraging mobility in the home environment, encouraging people to serve themselves drinks and snacks, providing opportunities to go outside, housework, domestic chores, shopping and gardening.

- **Recreational activities** can include hobbies such as cookery, gardening, pets, reading, woodwork, singing, treasure chest/rummage boxes with objects and memorabilia, poetry reading/recitation, dressing up, looking at large picture books or magazines, conversation starters to jog memories and conversation, listening to music favourites, helping with outings.

- **Relaxation activities** can involve a variety of techniques such as hand massage, a relaxation routine and listening to music. Pet therapy can also benefit health and well-being and many care settings bring in pets for residents to stroke, helping them to relax and form a bond.

- **Reminiscence** involves discussions (using props), inter-generational projects, outings, singing, links with local libraries, community organisations and schools, looking at life history books.

- **Sensory activities** involve using different textures and fabrics, exploring the smells of foods and perfumes, pets, personal care activities (using creams, oils and bubble baths) and music.

- **Social group activities** involve interaction and communication (both verbal and non-verbal) through smiling, laughing, practising social skills and behaviour. People can take part in games, quizzes, outings, tea dances and parties, sing together, bring in special occasion cakes/food, drink tea out of china cups, or have a sherry/ Baileys or drink of choice.

- **Spiritual activities** involve religious and cultural activities, music and singing.

Field Trips/Outings

In care settings such as nursing homes and day care centres, activities are regularly planned for clients by an activity co-ordinator. In nursing homes, these activities are usually scheduled in the afternoon or evening. Day trips or outings may also be organised.

These activities could include many of the activities listed above as well as dancing, bingo, swimming, exercise classes, ball games, gardening (indoor or outdoor), day trips and many more. Monthly or seasonal activities based around Easter, Christmas, Valentine's Day, etc. can be celebrated in a way that is inclusive and fun.

They can also involve leaving the care facility (if able) to go shopping, to a movie, a family member's or friend's home, or anywhere else the client(s) wants to go.

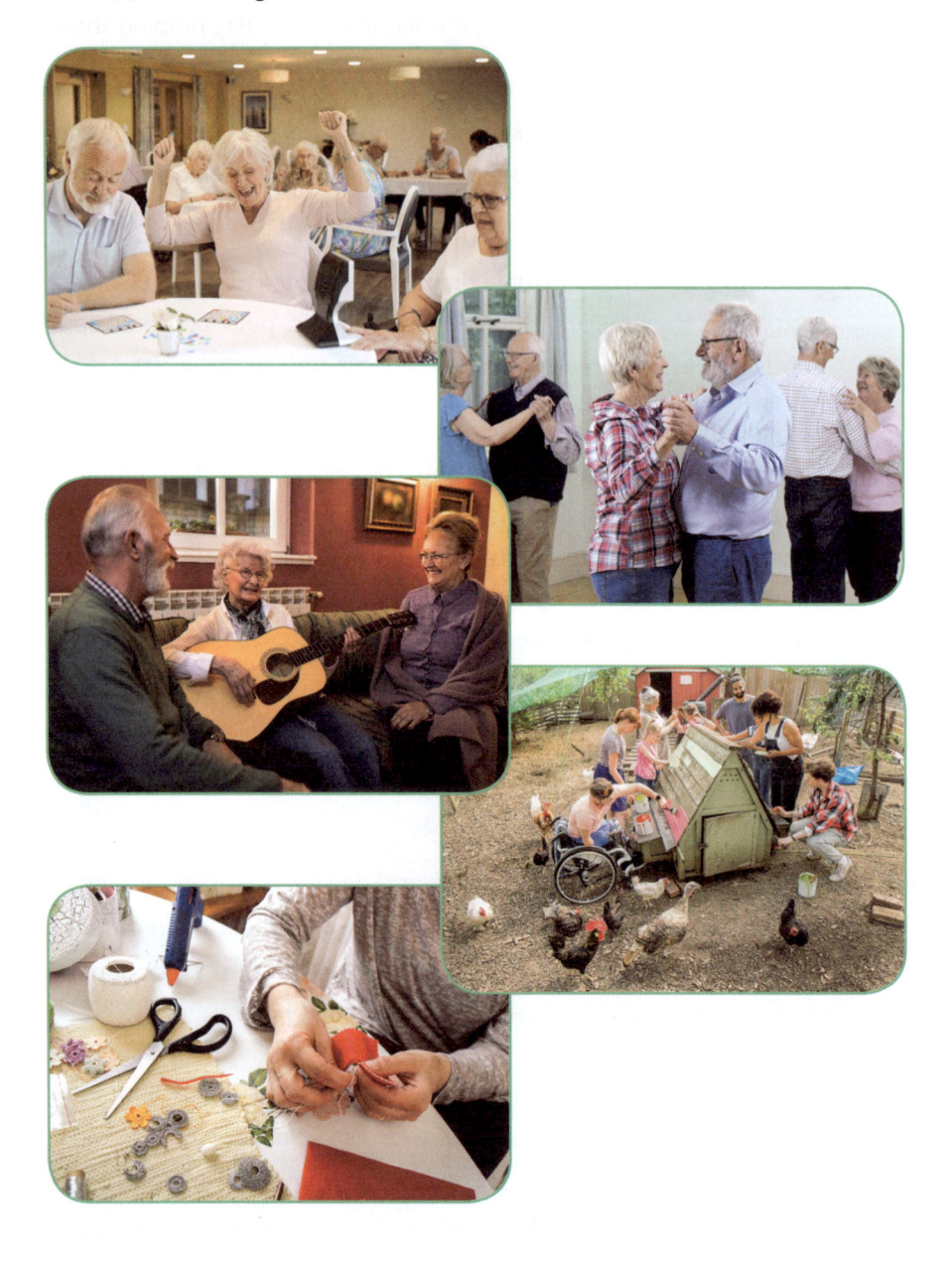

Activities Involving External Groups

+ **Oral history projects:** Groups such as Cuimhneamh an Chláir (Memories of Clare) gather the oral histories of older people. This is a valuable resource for future generations and a source of pleasure for those involved.

+ **Intergenerational projects:** These bring old and young people together, for example Transition Year students teaching older people how to use technology and social media. These projects benefit both groups, as skills are learned, and bonds are created between the young and old.

+ **Life story:** You could create a life story book with your clients. Include photos and any memorabilia that has meaning for the client. Contact the local library or historical society for background information and photos of past events to incorporate in a personal life story. Many older clients enjoy reminiscing and they can leave behind a lovely record of their lives.

> **Task** List some activities that you think would be suitable for clients in a care setting.

CULTURAL CONSIDERATIONS

Many of the holiday celebrations in Ireland, such as Christmas and Easter, are centred on the Christian religion. Confirm that your clients are happy to participate in these activities. If you are caring for clients from another culture or religion, do acknowledge their celebrations.

FITTING ACTIVITIES INTO YOUR DAILY ROUTINE

It can sometimes be hard to find time to include social activities in a busy working day, but social activities don't have to take much time.

If you have only **five minutes** you can use it to:

- talk to the clients and show an interest in them
- sit with them and read the newspaper
- encourage them to walk to the window and look out on the garden
- put on some music they like
- involve them in what you are doing, e.g. laying a table, tidying a room
- sing or hum a tune together
- encourage them to carry out some aspect of personal care, such as brushing their hair or teeth
- help them to select an album, scrapbook or book to look at
- share a poem, article or short story that you think they might like
- ask them if they'd like to listen to the radio or watch television
- stop for a moment to watch television together and talk about what you have seen
- put out different objects of interest in the communal room to explore and investigate each day
- create a multisensory environment for residents to interact with.

If you have only **15 minutes**, you can use it to:

- help residents start a game of cards, board game or word game
- read a newspaper or magazine together
- support a resident to attend a group or to start an activity
- go for a walk together, taking a turn round the garden

- invite residents to take their tea/coffee at the table rather than sitting in their chairs

- offer a hand massage, manicure or some other grooming activity

- support a resident to keep a scrapbook or photo album

- sit down with a resident to have a cup of tea or other refreshment

- support a resident to tell relatives and visitors about the news in the home

- help them to undertake small jobs, such as watering pot plants, refilling the bird feeder, delivering the post or newspapers

- help residents to look after and feed small animals, if available in the care setting

- read out loud a poem, article, or few pages of a story (RCOT 2015).

PLANNING AND PREPARATION

Prepare your activity well in advance. You must have a well-prepared timetable of events to avoid the activities running too short or too long and upsetting or tiring your clients. Make sure that your planned activity is suitable for your clients and their abilities. Prepare your equipment and make sure that you have enough for everyone. Determine how many carers are needed to help with the activity. Check all care plans and consult with your supervisor/nurse in charge.

- Select themes based on the residents' interests and experiences.

- Involve residents in the choice of theme.

- Be age-appropriate.

- Plan activities based on the residents' abilities and needs.

- Include an element of surprise and novelty to capture the imagination.

- Involve others in planning and collecting props.

- Abandon a theme that is uninspiring.

And, as always:

- **Prepare yourself:** Always attend to hand hygiene and assess whether PPE is needed.

- **Prepare the clients:** Introduce yourself, give explanations and gain consent.

- **Prepare the environment:** Furniture may need to be moved. Prepare your equipment and make sure that you have enough for everyone.

SAFETY

Safety is paramount throughout the activity, so prepare your environment, check your equipment and ensure that there are enough staff available to supervise and assist the clients. Make sure that equipment is safe.

After the activity, tidy everything and store equipment safely. Pay attention to good manual handling practice and hygiene.

AFTER THE ACTIVITY

- Assist clients as necessary, washing hands, removing any protective clothing, etc.

- Clean up all equipment.

- Return furniture to its original place.
- Display any work by the clients, with their consent.
- Attend to hand hygiene.
- Report and document the activity.

Task: Plan an activity or an outing that you think would be suitable for an individual or group of individuals who need care. The activity will need to be adapted to the needs of the individual(s).

Revision Questions:

1. What are the benefits of socialising for elderly people?
2. How can you encourage them to get involved?
3. How would you plan a social event or outing?
4. What can happen to a client who will not socialise or engage with others?
5. List five indoor and five outdoor activities that elderly people might enjoy or like to take part in.

Key words/phrases:

socialising

encouraging involvement

client's consent

independence

enjoyment

positive self-image

cognitive benefits

depression

SAFETY 13

The safety of the client and of the carer is paramount. There is a legal requirement to maintain the safety of all people in the workplace – workers, clients and visitors. The **Safety, Health and Welfare at Work Act 2005** emphasises the importance of safety in the workplace and focuses on the importance of preventing accidents. Prevention of accidents is the most important goal of safety and health in the workplace. Accidents can lead to pain, injury, loss of work days, loss of income, poor staff morale and, in the worst cases, death.

IN THIS CHAPTER YOU WILL LEARN ABOUT:

- Health and safety legislation
- Safety statements
- The importance of risk assessments
- The main health and safety issues in healthcare:
  - Manual handling
  - Slips and trips
  - Violence in the workplace

LEGISLATION

The Safety, Health and Welfare at Work Act 2005 sets out the importance of safety and health in the workplace. Accident prevention is a key goal, and under the act it is a legal requirement for the workplace to have a **safety statement**. This is a written document that sets out the safety measures that must be taken in the workplace. It is an action plan.

- It identifies any hazards in the workplace, i.e. anything that could cause an accident.

- Once the hazards are identified, a risk assessment needs to be carried out to determine how likely it is that the hazard will cause an accident. A risk may be low, medium or high.

- Once the risk assessment is carried out, the workplace should set out any control measures necessary to minimise the risk of an accident occurring.

- The safety statement should also set out any procedures to be followed in the event of an emergency, such as evacuation due to fire. It should name any persons with responsibility for health and safety in the workplace.

The Safety, Health and Welfare at Work (Chemical Agents) Regulations 2001 and the Safety, Health and Welfare at Work (Chemical Agents) (Amendment) Regulations 2015 require employers to take actions to prevent or significantly reduce their workers' exposure to any substances that would be hazardous to their health.

RISK MANAGEMENT

Risk management is a three-step process:

1. **Hazard identification:** Identifying the hazards – anything that can cause harm – associated with the workplace and the work activities. Hazards can be physical, chemical, biological or human factor.

    - *Physical hazards* include manual handling activities; equipment that has been poorly maintained, is used incorrectly or not suitable for the task; slipping and tripping hazards such as wet or poorly maintained floors.

- *Chemical hazards* are chemical substances such as cleaning, disinfecting or sterilising agents, medical gases, etc.

- *Biological hazards* include viruses and bacteria that can cause infection, e.g. exposure to blood and body fluids; exposure to airborne pathogens such as tuberculosis and Legionnaires' disease.

- *Human factor hazards:* people should be mentally and physically capable of doing their job. The workplace, the work system, the organisation of work and the job should be designed so as to avoid causing sustained stress, such as bullying, harassment and violence.

2. **Risk assessment:** Assessing risk involves estimating how likely it is that a hazard will cause harm, how serious that harm is likely to be, how often and how many people are exposed and what control measures are already in place.

3. **Controls:** If there are safety measures already in place, the risk assessment will clearly indicate whether they are adequate. When a risk to staff is uncovered, a solution or precaution must be implemented to control the risk. Risk assessments should be reviewed and updated regularly (HSA 2010).

MANUAL HANDLING

Manual handling carries the risk of injury to the musculoskeletal system. Most commonly, the back is affected. The Health and Safety Authority define manual handling as involving any transporting or supporting of any load by one or more employees, and it includes lifting, putting down, pushing, pulling, carrying or moving a load, **which by reason of its**

characteristics or unfavourable ergonomic conditions, involves risk, particularly of back injury, to employees (HSA 2011).

Patient handling carries a particular risk because they are an unpredictable load; they may not co-operate with you when handling them.

Points to remember when carrying out manual handling:

- Carers must have up-to-date training in manual and patient handling and follow the manual handling guidelines.
- Assess the risk – TILE (Task, Individual, Load, Environment); see below.
- It is advisable that carers work in pairs (though this is not always necessary).
- Use manual handling aids, e.g. hoist, handling belts, transfer boards, etc.
- Follow the principles of safe lifting.
- Encourage the clients to move themselves, if possible.
- Report any accidents or near-misses.

Employers are legally bound to provide continuous up-to-date manual handling training to all staff in the healthcare setting, who may find themselves in the position where manual handling knowledge is required.

TILE Risk Assessment

Task: This includes requirements of the activity such as excessive lifting, lowering or carrying distances and physical effort.

> **Individual:** The individual's physical capability, training and knowledge.
>
> **Load:** The characteristics of a load – which can be either an object or a person – such as weight, size, difficulty of grasping, etc.
>
> **Environment:** Available space, uneven or slippery floors, unsuitable temperature, etc. (HSE 2011).

Principles of Safe Lifting

- Assess the task – the area and load.
- Work from a broad, stable base (feet flat on the floor).
- Bend the knees.
- Keep the back straight – not necessarily vertical.
- Keep a firm grip with the palm of the hand (palmar grip).
- Keep arms in line with trunk.
- Keep weight close to the centre of gravity.
- Turn the feet in the direction of movement.

SLIPS AND TRIPS IN THE HEALTHCARE SETTING

The workplace can be a hazardous place, with wet and slippery floors and clutter that can create tripping hazards. Clients who are frail and unsteady on their feet are particularly at risk. The carer should take all precautions to prevent the workers and the clients from slipping or tripping.

To minimise the risk:

- Assess the work area.
- Make room by moving furniture before performing cares.
- Take care when washing to avoid spillages.
- Clean up any spillages immediately.
- Avoid clutter.
- Ensure that there is ample storage for clients' belongings.
- Avoid trailing leads or cables.
- Report any accidents or near misses.

RESPONDING TO CHALLENGING BEHAVIOUR

The vulnerable and unpredictable character of some clients means that carers are at risk of being exposed to violence, either verbal or physical. Verbal violence can include being shouted at, insulted or threatened. Physical violence could be a scrape, a pinch, a bite or a more serious assault. Violence in the workplace can be very distressing and all carers are entitled to feel safe in their workplace.

The carer must be aware of the clients they are looking after. A client who is suffering from dementia, mental illness or an intellectual disability may not be responsible for their actions; others may be feeling anxious, threatened and afraid. However, it is important to remember that not all clients living with dementia, mental illness or an intellectual disability are violent. Each client must be assessed individually.

To minimise the risk of violence in the workplace:

+ Assess the risk – some workplaces have a higher risk of violence than others and some clients are at a higher risk of being violent than others.

+ Education and training can help the workers to deal with violent clients or challenging behaviour.

+ Be aware of triggers to aggression and warning cues.

+ Modify your behaviour to reduce the risk of further aggravating a violent client. Speak in a calm voice and behave in a calm manner. Avoid a sharp voice and sudden movements.

+ Avoid confrontation.

+ Distract the client if possible.

+ Ensure that there are adequate staffing levels – work in pairs, avoid being alone with a client who is at risk of becoming violent.

+ Report incidents or near misses.

+ Seek help if you are feeling distressed following an incident.

De-escalation Techniques

The effective handling of a challenging or aggressive situation is very demanding. This is one area where good interaction and communication skills are required. Communication is about listening, hearing and speaking, as well as body language and non-verbal interaction.

Here are some de-escalation techniques:

+ Defuse the situation.

+ Stay calm and appear confident.

- Create some space.
- Lower your voice.
- Avoid confrontation, threats or ultimatums.
- Negotiate; use open questions.
- Remove yourself from the situation/provide time-out for the person.

> Training is mandatory to ensure adequate care is taken when engaging in manual handling, ensuring infection prevention and control (discussed in Chapter 11), when promoting prevention of slips and trips and if exposed to challenging behaviour.

Reporting

It is important to document and report any incident that occurs in the workplace that compromises the health and safety of both carer and client. The relevant forms must be completed and presented to your supervisor. An **ABC Chart** (see Appendix 8) helps record information about behaviour.

ABC Chart

An ABC chart is an observational tool that allows us to record information about a particular behaviour to better understand what the behaviour is communicating.

- **A – the antecedent:** The event that occurred before the behaviour was exhibited. This can include what the person was doing; who was there and where they were; the sights, sounds, smells, temperatures in the environment; the number of people who were in the environment.

- **B – behaviour:** An objective and clear description of the behaviour that occurred, e.g. X threw item on the floor.

> **+ C – consequence:** What occurred after the behaviour, or the consequence of the behaviour, e.g. noise levels in the room decreased.
>
> It is important to decide on one or two target behaviours to record initially. Place the ABC chart in an accessible place to make it easier to use after the target behaviour has been exhibited (RVCPH: n.d.).

STAFF IMMUNISATION

A high level of personal hygiene and appropriate immunisations provide good baseline protection for carers against the spread of infections. The National Immunisation Advisory Committee recommends specific vaccinations for healthcare workers who have significant client contact:

- **Hepatitis B:** You should get immunised against hepatitis B infection if you are at risk of contact with blood, body fluids or at risk of needle stick injury.

- **Influenza:** The flu vaccine is offered to all healthcare staff during the influenza season each year.

- **TB skin test:** This is not an immunisation, but a pre-employment skin test is recommended if you have no evidence of a BCG scar or no documented evidence of having received a BCG vaccination.

- **Measles/mumps/rubella:** A blood test will be taken to check for immunity for those born before 1978. If non-immune, two doses of MMR are recommended. For people born after 1978, evidence of two MMR vaccines will be required.

- **Varicella:** A blood test will be taken to check immunity. If non-immune, vaccination will be offered (HSE 2011).

CHAPTER 13: SAFETY

> **Task:** Perform a risk assessment of the hazards in your workplace. Suggest control measures to reduce the risk of an accident occurring.

Revision Questions:

1. What is the main legislation governing health and safety in the workplace?
2. What are the three steps in risk management?
3. Why is manual handling training so important?
4. What is a safety statement?

Key words/phrases:

Safety, Health and Welfare at Work Act 2005

safety statement

manual handling

risk management

hazard identification

assessing risk

reporting incidents

staff immunisation

slips and trips

challenging behaviour

ABC chart

REPORTING AND DOCUMENTATION

14

As a carer you will need to pass on important information to the nurse in charge or your supervisor. You must know what needs to be reported and how to report. Some things need to be reported urgently; others can be reported after cares have been given. Carers are also involved in documenting cares, either handwritten or electronic. The carer needs to be aware of the importance of careful and accurate documentation.

> **IN THIS CHAPTER YOU WILL LEARN ABOUT:**
> - Why you should report
> - What you should report
> - How you should report
> - Examples of client documentation

WHAT SHOULD YOU REPORT?

You need to have good communication with your supervisor. It is important to report any changes or concerns to the supervisor. The carer is responsible for many of the day-to-day observations on a client. In some settings, such as a nursing home, there may be only one or two qualified nurses on duty, so the carer needs to be aware of any changes in the client that need reporting – changes in their condition may be a sign that there is something seriously wrong.

You must report:

- Changes in vital signs, such as low or high temperature, high or low blood pressure, changes in pulse or respiratory rate.
- Changes in eating and drinking habits, for example the client refusing food.
- Changes in bowel habits.
- Changes in urinary output.
- Changes in mood.
- Changes in sleeping pattern.
- Cognitive changes, e.g. signs of confusion or forgetfulness.
- Significant weight loss or weight gain.
- Changes to skin integrity.
- Changes to level of independence.
- Visual changes – if the client looks unwell.
- Bruising or injuries.
- Accidents or incidents.

> **Task** Can you think of anything else that you should report?

If you feel that the client is 'not themselves', but you are not sure why, it is always best to report this. Carers spend a lot of time with their clients and are often the first to notice any deterioration in condition.

HOW DO YOU REPORT?

Information passed on to your supervisor must be **clear** and **specific**, e.g. 'Mrs Brown in Room 12 has not had any breakfast today, but she normally has a good appetite. She said she is not feeling well and she looks pale.'

If it is an emergency, the information must be passed on **immediately**. For example, if you find a client has collapsed and you are on your own, first make sure that the environment is safe (always look out for your safety), then call out for help. If a co-worker is with you, send them to get the nurse in charge. Calmly give your co-worker clear instructions, e.g. 'Go to the office and ask Mary to come quickly. Tell her that Jack Smith has collapsed by his bed in Room 6.'

ACCIDENT REPORTING

All accidents in the workplace must be reported and an incident form completed. The information that must be recorded on an incident form includes:

- the details of the person involved in the accident
- the details of any witnesses
- the details of the incident – where, when, how, what. Put in as much detail as possible, stick to the facts, avoid judgemental language
- if there is an injury and the nature of the injury
- if the client has received medical attention.

The form must be signed, and in some settings it must also be signed by the client's next of kin.

CLIENT DOCUMENTATION

In some workplaces carers are responsible for completing written documentation detailing the cares given. The purpose of documentation is that it allows continuity of care. It contains information about the cares given to the client so that the care staff who come on duty after you can see what cares have been given and what needs to be done. It is evidence of the cares given.

Documentation must be written clearly and must be legible. Use a black pen for written documentation and include the time, the date and your signature. Abbreviations should be avoided, although some workplaces have agreed abbreviations that may be used. It should be non-judgemental and objective – stick to the facts. It should be relevant.

> If you make a mistake when you are documenting information, do not use Tipp-Ex. Draw a line through the error, print and sign your name and write the date and time. Include details about the reason for the correction. Documentation of cares should be done as soon as possible after giving the cares when the information will be fresh in your mind.

Types of Client Documentation

- **Care plans:** These set out the cares given to the client during your work shift. In some settings a computerised system such as EpicCare is used. Care plans need to be completed at the end of every work shift.

- **Food intake chart** (see Appendix 1): All food and drink the client has taken in.

- **Fluid Balance Chart (fluid intake and output)** (see Appendix 2): Fluid input and output over a 24-hour period.

- **Pressure sore risk assessment chart**, e.g. a Waterlow chart (see Appendix 3).

- **Observation charts** (see Appendix 5): Record blood pressure, pulse, temperature and rate of respiration.

- **Turns chart** (see Appendix 4): How often the client has been turned.

- **Falls risk assessment** (see Appendix 5): Assesses if the client is at risk of falling.

- **Mood chart** (see Appendix 6): The client's moods throughout the day.

- **Pain scores** (see Appendix 7): Usually scored from most severe to no pain at all.

- **ABC chart** (see Appendix 8): An observational tool that records information about a particular behaviour.

- **Nutritional assessment** (see Appendix 9): Assesses if the client is well nourished.

Exercise:

Diane Bates is an 86-year-old resident in Shady Oak Nursing Home. She has arthritis and diabetes and mobilises with a Zimmer frame and supervision.

At 10 p.m., while you were with another client, you witnessed Diane climb out of bed and try to walk to the bathroom. Her Zimmer frame was stored at the end of the bed and she couldn't reach it. She slipped and fell at the end of the bed. She injured her left leg in the fall and had a cut to her forehead.

- Fill in the incident form on the next page.

Shady Oak Nursing Home

INCIDENT REPORT FORM

Name of person involved in accident: _____

Address: _____

_____

Ward: _____

Nurse in charge: _____

Date of occurrence: _____

Time of occurrence: _____

Where did the incident occur? _____

Full description of incident: _____

_____

_____

_____

_____

_____

Details of injuries suffered: _____

_____

_____

Name of doctor or hospital attended: _____

Any follow-up actions to reduce possibility of re-occurrence:

_____

_____

Witnesses: _____

_____

Signature: _____

Date: _____

COMPLETE CARE SKILLS

Revision Questions:

1. Why is recording and reporting so important?
2. List five things you should always report.
3. How should you deal with an error on a report?

Key words/phrases:

reporting

client documentation

care plans

observation chart

fluid balance chart

food chart

mood chart

pain scores

turns chart

pressure sores assessment chart (Waterlow chart)

falls risk assessment chart

nutrition chart

END OF LIFE CARE

15

Sometimes the person you are caring for has an illness that cannot be cured. Eventually this illness may result in death. You may have to care for that person at the end of their life and you will need to consider the following cares as part of your routine.

> **IN THIS CHAPTER YOU WILL LEARN ABOUT END OF LIFE CARE, FOCUSING ON:**
>
> - A Client's Comfort and Personal Care
> - Pain Management
> - Pressure Sores
> - Meeting Nutritional Needs
> - Communication
> - Family Care
> - Cultural Needs
> - Loss and Grief
> - The Five Stages of Grief

Client's Comfort and Personal Care

When caring for a person at the end of their life you want to keep the person comfortable. You will try to make the person's final days as good as possible for both the client and their family and help the person to die peacefully. It is important that you keep the client comfortable. Reposition them and support them with pillows. If the patient has trouble breathing, help him or her to sit up a little.

Keep the client clean and comfortable. Assist with washing. Clean the eyes if they have secretions. Attend to oral care and keep lips moistened.

Pain Management

The person at the end of their life is likely to be in pain and will be on painkillers. Be aware of some of the side effects of the painkillers and report any concerns to your supervisor/nurse in charge. Some medications can cause constipation, nausea, sleepiness, hallucinations or twitching. You can help the client deal with their pain by keeping them comfortable. Massage, music or a hot pad can help the client control their pain.

Pressure Sores

Check the skin, as a client requiring end-of-life care is at risk of getting pressure sores. Help the client get out of bed and sit in a chair if they are able. If not, change their position every two hours and try to keep the patient in whatever positions are most comfortable.

Meeting Nutritional Needs

At the end of a person's life they have less need for food and drink. It is normal for a person who is dying not to feel like eating or drinking. Eating and drinking becomes more of an effort for them. They might need help to take sips of fluid. A drinking beaker or straw can make this easier. Moistening their lips and tongue with water or oral gel helps keep them comfortable.

Communication

Communicate with the client. Continue to speak to them and explain all procedures. Even when clients are close to death, they can hear, so do not speak in a whisper – speak clearly. The client will also still feel your touch.

Family Care

Care for the family too. Their needs are also important, and you will also provide comfort to the family. The family are not restricted to visiting hours when their relative is at the end of their life. Make sure that they are comfortable and feel welcome. Where possible, include them in the client's cares.

Cultural Needs

Be aware of any cultural or religious needs of the client. Ask the client and their family. They may wish to be visited by a priest, rabbi, imam or the equivalent person in their religion.

After Death

When the client has died, allow the family to be with them. Follow the guidelines of your workplace for laying out the client, which involves washing and dressing the body.

LOSS AND GRIEF

When you care for a client who is at the end of their life or who dies, you must recognise that this may affect you emotionally.

The Five Stages of Grief

When a client dies you may experience feelings of loss and grief. You will have built up a relationship and a bond with this person. You may find it helps to talk about these feelings with your work colleagues. They are likely to share your feelings.

Elisabeth Kübler-Ross identified five stages of grief:

- Denial: a refusal to believe that they are dying
- Anger: 'Why me?'
- Bargaining: maybe bargaining with God for more time, usually done privately
- Depression: mourning over things that are lost
- Acceptance of death: calmness and peace.

You may see the person you are caring for go through these five stages as they deal with their journey towards death. You will also experience many of these feelings of grief after the person has died (Marie Curie: Palliative Care Knowledge Zone).

Revision Questions:

1. How can you make a client comfortable during end of life care?
2. What are the five stages of grief?

Key words/phrases:

loss

five stages of grief

Appendices

APPENDIX 1: EXAMPLE OF A FOOD INTAKE CHART

Date:	Description of food and drink provided	Portion size provided			Amount taken					Fluid consumed (ml)	Action and signature
		S	M	L	None	¼	½	¾	All		
Breakfast											
Mid-morning											
Lunch											
Mid-afternoon											
Tea											
Supper											
Night time											
Total fluids consumed in 24 hours:											

APPENDIX 2: EXAMPLE OF A FLUID BALANCE CHART (FLUID INTAKE AND OUTPUT)

Fluid Balance Chart				Name:				
Room:				Date of Birth:				
INTAKE				OUTPUT				
Time - 24 Hour	Intra-venous	Peg Nutrition	Oral	Vomit	Urine	Bowel	Stoma

APPENDIX 3: WATERLOW CHART

WATERLOW PRESSURE ULCER PREVENTION/ TREATMENT POLICY

Ring scores in table, add total. More than 1 score/category can be used.
Source: http://www.judy-waterlow.co.uk

BUILD/ WEIGHT FOR HEIGHT	♦	SKIN TYPE VISUAL RISK AREAS	♦	SEX AGE	♦	MALNUTRITION SCREENING TOOL (MST)		
Average BMI = 20–24.9	0	Healthy	0	MALE	1	**A** HAS PATIENT LOST WEIGHT RECENTLY? YES – GO TO B NO – GO TO C UNSURE – GO TO C AND SCORE 2	**B** WEIGHT LOSS SCORE 0.5–5kg = 1 5–10kg = 2 10–15kg = 3 > 15kg = 4 Unsure = 2	
Above Average BMI = 25–29.9	1	Tissue Paper	1	FEMALE	2			
Obese BMI > 30	2	Dry	1	14–49	1			
Below Average BMI > 20	3	Oedema-tous	1	50–64	2			
BMI = Wt (kg)/Ht (m)		Clammy, Pyrexia	1	65–74	3			
		Dis-coloured Grade 1	2	75–80	4			
				81+	5			
CONTINENCE	♦	Broken spots Grade 2–4	3			**C** PATIENT EATING POORLY OR LACK OF APPETITE NO = 0 YES = Score = 1	NUTRITION SCORE If > 2 refer for nutrition assessment/ intervention	
Complete/ Catheter-ised	0							
Urine incont.	1	MOBILITY	♦	**SPECIAL RISKS**				
Faecal incont.	2	Fully	0	TISSUE MALNUTRITION		♦	NEUROLOGICAL DEFICIT	♦
Urinary + Faecal incon-tinence	3	Restless/ Fidgety	1	TERMINAL CACHEXIA		8	DIABETES, MS, CVA	4–6
		Apathetic	2	MULTIPLE ORGAN FAILURE		8	MOTOR/SENSORY PARAPLEGIA (MAX. OF 6)	4–6 4–6
		Restricted	3	SINGLE ORGAN FAILURE (RESP, RENAL, CARDIAC)		5		
SCORE		Bedbound e.g. Traction	4				**MAJOR SURGERY OR TRAUMA**	
10+ AT RISK		Chair-bound e.g. Wheel-chair	5	PERIPHERAL VASCULAR DISEASE		5	ORTHOPAEDIC/ SPINAL	5
15+ HIGH RISK				ANAEMIA (Hb < 8)		2	ON TABLE > 2 hrs	5
20+ VERY HIGH RISK				SMOKING		1	ON TABLE < 6 hrs	8
				MEDICATION – CYTOTOXICS, LONG-TERM/HIGH-DOSE STEROIDS, ANTI-INFLAMMATORY MAX. OF 4				

APPENDIX 4: EXAMPLE OF A TURNS CHART

Date: _____

TIME	PATIENT'S POSITION	COMMENTS	SIGNATURE	TIME	PATIENT'S POSITION	COMMENTS	SIGNATURE
01:00				13:00			
02:00				14:00			
03:00				15:00			
04:00				16:00			
05:00				17:00			
06:00				18:00			
07:00				19:00			
08:00				20:00			
09:00				21:00			
10:00				22:00			
11:00				23:00			
12:00				24:00			

KEY:

PATIENT'S POSITION

(M) Patient mobilising   *Change patient's position

(L) Left side _____ hourly

(R) Right side

(P) Prone

(B) Back

(C) To sit out in armchair   * Patient can sit in armchair

(T) Therapy (physio, OT) for _____ hour only

(I) Investigation (Imaging dept)

APPENDIX 5: EXAMPLE OF AN OBSERVATION CHART

Reproduced from: Royal College of Physicians. National Early Warning Score (NEWS) 2: Standardising the assessment of acute-illness severity in the NHS. Updated report of a working party. London: RCP, 2017.

APPENDIX 6: EXAMPLE OF A MOOD CHART

MOOD CHART

NAME:
DATE:
ROOM:

TIME	HAPPY	SAD	MAD	TIRED	EXCITED	WORRIED	SCARED	OTHER	NOTES
6-8									
8-10									
10-12									
12-2									
2-4									
4-6									
6-8									
8-10									
10-12									
12-2									
2-4									
4-6									

APPENDIX 7: EXAMPLE OF A FALLS RISK ASSESSMENT CHART

FALL RISK ASSESSMENT CHART		
Client Name:		Doctor:
Room:	Assesor:	Date:

KEY

Low Risk	Moderate Risk	High Risk

Category	Characteristic	1 (Assessment Date #1)	2 (Assessment Date #1)	3 (Assessment Date #1)	4 (Assessment Date #1)	Evaluation
Fall History	NO FALLS in past 3 months					
	1–2 FALLS in past 3 months					
	3 OR MORE FALLS in past 3 months					
Medications	*Respond below based on these mediations: anesthetics, antihistamines, antihypertensives, antiseizures, benzodiazepines, cathartics, diuretics, hypoglycemics, narcotics, psychotropics, sedatives/hypnotics*					
	Currently takes none of these medications					
	Currently takes 1–2 of these medications					
	Currently takes 3–4 of these medications					
	A change in medication and/or dosage in past 5 days					
Continence Status	Ambulatory/continent					
	Wheelchair or ambulatory aid/continent					
	Ambulatory/incontent					
	Wheelchair or ambulatory aid/incontinent					
Vision/ Hearing	Adequate (with or without glasses/hearing aid)					
	Poor (with or without glasses/hearing aid)					
	Legally Blind or very hard of hearing/deaf					
Predisposing Diseases/ Conditions	*Respond below based on these conditions: hypotension, vertigo, CVA, Parkinson's, loss of limb(s), seizures, arthritis, osteoporosis, fractures, dementia, delirium, anemia, wandering, anger*					
	None present					
	1–2 present					
	3 or more present					

APPENDIX 8: EXAMPLE OF AN ABC CHART

Date/Time	Activity	Antecedent	Behaviour	Consequence
Date/time when the behaviour occurred	What activity was going on when the behaviour occurred	What happened just before the behaviour that *might* have triggered the behaviour	What the behaviour looked like	What happened after the behaviour, or as a result of the behaviour

APPENDIX 9: MINI NUTRITIONAL ASSESSMENT

Mini Nutritional Assessment MNA®

Nestlé NutritionInstitute

Last name: _____ First name: _____
Sex: _____ Age: _____ Weight, kg: _____ Height, cm: _____ Date: _____

Complete the screen by filling in the boxes with the appropriate numbers. Total the numbers for the final screening score.

Screening

A Has food intake declined over the past 3 months due to loss of appetite, digestive problems, chewing or swallowing difficulties?
0 = severe decrease in food intake
1 = moderate decrease in food intake
2 = no decrease in food intake ☐

B Weight loss during the last 3 months
0 = weight loss greater than 3 kg (6.6 lbs)
1 = does not know
2 = weight loss between 1 and 3 kg (2.2 and 6.6 lbs)
3 = no weight loss ☐

C Mobility
0 = bed or chair bound
1 = able to get out of bed / chair but does not go out
2 = goes out ☐

D Has suffered psychological stress or acute disease in the past 3 months?
0 = yes   2 = no ☐

E Neuropsychological problems
0 = severe dementia or depression
1 = mild dementia
2 = no psychological problems ☐

F1 Body Mass Index (BMI) (weight in kg) / (height in m)^2
0 = BMI less than 19
1 = BMI 19 to less than 21
2 = BMI 21 to less than 23
3 = BMI 23 or greater ☐

IF BMI IS NOT AVAILABLE, REPLACE QUESTION F1 WITH QUESTION F2.
DO NOT ANSWER QUESTION F2 IF QUESTION F1 IS ALREADY COMPLETED.

F2 Calf circumference (CC) in cm
0 = CC less than 31
3 = CC 31 or greater ☐

Screening score (max. 14 points)

12 - 14 points: Normal nutritional status
8 - 11 points: At risk of malnutrition
0 - 7 points: Malnourished ☐☐

References
1. Vellas B, Villars H, Abellan G, et al. Overview of the MNA® - Its History and Challenges. *J Nutr Health Aging.* 2006;**10**:456-465.
2. Rubenstein LZ, Harker JO, Salva A, Guigoz Y, Vellas B. Screening for Undernutrition in Geriatric Practice: Developing the Short-Form Mini Nutritional Assessment (MNA-SF). *J. Geront.* 2001; **56A**: M366-377
3. Guigoz Y. The Mini-Nutritional Assessment (MNA®) Review of the Literature - What does it tell us? *J Nutr Health Aging.* 2006; **10**:466-487.
4. Kaiser MJ, Bauer JM, Ramsch C, et al. Validation of the Mini Nutritional Assessment Short-Form (MNA®-SF): A practical tool for identification of nutritional status. *J Nutr Health Aging.* 2009; **13**:782-788.

® Société des Produits Nestlé, S.A., Vevey, Switzerland, Trademark Owners © Nestlé, 1994, Revision 2009. N67200 12/99 10M
For more information: www.mna-elderly.com

Source: www.mna-elderly.com/forms/MNA_english.pdf

REFERENCES

Association of Occupational Therapists of Ireland (AOTI) (website) <www.aoti.ie>

Back, A., Arnold, R. and Tulsky, J. (2009). *Mastering Communication with Seriously Ill Patients: Balancing honesty with empathy and hope*. Cambridge University Press.

Barbour, V., Clark, J., Jones, S. and Veitch, E. (2010). *Social Relationships Are Key to Health, and to Health Policy*. PLoS Med 7(8): e1000334. https://doi.org/10.1371/journal.pmed.1000334

Careers Portal (website). 'General Nurse (RGN)' <https://careersportal.ie/careers/detail.php?job_id=315>

Health Information and Quality Authority (HIQA) (2012). *A Guide to the National Standards for Safer Better Healthcare*. Dublin: HIQA.

Health and Safety Authority (HSA) (2010). *Health and Safety Management in Healthcare*. Dublin: HSA. <https://www.hsa.ie/eng/Publications_and_Forms/Publications/Healthcare_Sector/Health_and_Safety_Management_in_Healthcare.pdf>

Health and Safety Authority (HSA) (2010). *Health and Safety at Work in Residential Care Facilities* <https://www.hsa.ie/eng/Publications_and_Forms/Publications/Healthcare_Sector/Residential_Care_Facilities.pdf>

https://www.hsa.ie/eng/Publications_and_Forms/Publications/Healthcare_Sector/Residential_Care_Facilities.pdf

— (2011). *Guidance on the Management of Manual Handling in Healthcare*. Dublin: HSA. <www.hsa.ie/eng/Publications_and_Forms/Publications/Healthcare_Sector/Manual_Handling_Health_Care.pdf>

Health Service Executive (HSE) (2006). *National Cleaning Manual Appendices*. Dublin: HSE.

— (2009). *Health Services: Intercultural Guide*. Dublin: HSE. <https://www.hse.ie/eng/services/publications/socialinclusion/interculturalguide/interculturalguide.pdf>

— (2011). *Infection Prevention and Control: An Information Booklet for Home Helps and Personal Assistants*. HSE South. <www.hse.ie/eng/about/who/healthwellbeing/infectcont/sth/gl/ipcc-guidelines-section-4>

— (2010). *Preventing Falls – Information Leaflet.* <www.hse.ie/eng/services/publications/olderpeople/preventing-falls---information-leaflet.pdf>.

— (2012a). *Special Geriatric Services Model of Care.* <www.hse.ie/eng/services/publications/clinical-strategy-and-programmes/specialist-geriatric-services-model-of-care.pdf>

— (2012b). 'Service User Falls Prevention in Healthcare: Think ACE!'. Dublin: HSE.

— (2018a). *Manual Handling and People Handling Policy*. Dublin: HSE. <www.hse.ie/eng/staff/safetywellbeing/healthsafetyand%20wellbeing/manualhandlingandpeoplehandlingpolicy.pdf>

— (2018b). *National Wound Management Guidelines*. Dublin: HSE. <https://www.hse.ie/eng/services/publications/nursingmidwifery%20services/wound-management-guidelines-2018.pdf>

- (n.d.) '"Hello my name is ..." Checklist for Implementation'. <www.hse.ie/eng/about/who/qid/person-family-engagement/hellomynameis/checklist-to-assist-hse-sites-implementin-hello-my-name-is-.pdf>

- (website) 'Bed Sores'. < www.hse.ie/eng/health/az/b/bed-sores/causes-of-pressure-ulcers.html>

- (website) 'Continence Promotion'. <www.hse.ie/eng/services/list/4/olderpeople/tipsforhealthyliving/continencepromotion.html#Managing%20incontinence>

- (website) 'Guidelines on Accessible Health and Social Care Services Guideline 4: Communication'. <http://www.hse.ie/eng/services/yourhealthservice/access/natguideaccessibleservices/part1.html#comm4>

- (website) 'Health and Wellbeing: Section 3 Standard Precautions'. <https://www.hse.ie/eng/about/who/healthwellbeing/infectcont/sth/gl/sec3.html>

- (website) 'Prevention of Pressure Ulcers'. <https://www.hse.ie/eng/about/who/qid/nationalsafetyprogrammes/pressureulcerszero/tissueviabilitypressureulcer.pdf>

Irish Society of Chartered Physiotherapists (ISCP) (website). 'What is Physiotherapy?' <www.iscp.ie/why-choose-chartered/what-is-physiotherapy>

Marie Curie (website). Palliative Care Knowledge Zone <https://www.mariecurie.org.uk/professionals/palliative-care-knowledge-zone>

Maslow, A.H. (1987). *Motivation and Personality* (3rd edn). Delhi, India: Pearson Education.

Mehrabian, A. (1981). *Silent messages: Implicit communication of emotions and attitudes.* Belmont, CA: Wadsworth.

McCance (DPhil, MSc, BSc Hons, Tanya & McCormack, Brendan & Dewing, Jan. (2011). *An Exploration of Person-Centredness in Practice. Online Journal of Issues in Nursing.* 16. 1. 10.3912/OJIN. Vol16No02Man01

Regional Virtual Classroom for Public Health (RVCPH) (n.d.). 'How to Use an ABC Chart'. <https://cursos.campusvirtualsp.org/pluginfile.php/87023/mod_resource/content/1/ABC%20Chart.pdf>

Roper, N., Logan, W.W. and Tierney A.J. (2000). *The Roper-Logan-Tierney Model of Nursing: Based on Activities of Living.* Edinburgh: Elsevier Health Sciences.

Royal College of Occupational Therapists (RCOT) (2015). *Living Well through Activity in Care Homes: The Toolkit.* London: RCOT. <https://www.rcot.co.uk/practice-resources/rcot-publications/downloads/living-well-care-homes>

Royal College of Physicians in Ireland (RCPI) Clinical Advisory Group on Healthcare Associated Infections and HSE Quality Improvement Division (2012). *Guidelines for Hand Hygiene in Irish Healthcare Settings.* Dublin: RCPI/HSE.

Sealy, Pat (2011). 'The power of empathy'. *Canadian Nurse*, October. <www.canadian-nurse.com/articles/issues/2011/october-2011/the-power-of-empathy>

Troyer, Angela K. (2016). 'The health benefits of socializing'. *Psychology Today*, 30 June. <www.psychologytoday.com/us/blog/living-mild-cognitive-impairment/201606/the-health-benefits-socializing>

World Health Organization (WHO) (1946). Constitution. <https://www.who.int/about/mission/en/>

BIBLIOGRAPHY

Townsend, K., *Fundamental Concepts and Skills for the Patient Care Technician*. Mosby, Missouri (2017).

Carter, Pamela J., *Lippincott's Textbook for Nursing Assistants: A Humanistic Approach to Caregiving*. Wolters Kluwer Health, Lippincott Williams & Wilkins, Iphen aan den Rijn (2012) (3rd edition).

Sorrentino, Sheila A., PhD RN, Remmert Leighann MS RN, *Mosby's Textbook for Nursing Assistants*. Mosby, Missouri (2016) (9th Edition).

Maslow, A. H., *Motivation and Personality*. Delhi, India: Pearson Education (1987) (3rd edition).

Nifast, *Care Skills & Care Support*. Dublin: Gill Education (2013).

USEFUL WEBSITES

Alzheimer Society of Ireland – www.alzheimer.ie

Assist Ireland Information on Daily Living Aids – www.assistireland.ie

Association of Occupational Therapists of Ireland (AOTI) – www.aoti.ie

Autism Ireland – www.autismireland.ie

Bord Bia Irish Food Board – www.bordbia.ie

Coeliac Society of Ireland – www.coeliac.ie

Cystic Fibrosis Ireland – www.cfireland.ie

Dementia Understand Together – www.understandtogether.ie

Diabetes Ireland – www.diabetes.ie

Health Information and Quality Authority (HIQA) – www.hiqa.ie

Health and Safety Authority (HSA) – www.hsa.ie

Health Service Executive (HSE) – www.hse.ie

Irish Hospice Foundation – www.hospicefoundation.ie

Irish Nutrition and Dietetic Institute (IDI) - www.indi.ie

Irish Osteoporosis Society – www.irishosteoporosis.ie

Irish Society of Chartered Physiotherapists (ISCP) – www.iscp.ie

Judy Waterlow Co. – www.judy-waterlow.co.uk

Marie Curie – www.mariecurie.org.uk

Royal College of Occupational Therapists (RCOT) – www.rcot.co.uk

World Health Organization (WHO) – www.who.int

INDEX

Abbreviations 171
Accidents 116 138 158 159 161 163 169 170
   Injuries 18 116 123 147 169
ACE (Assess, Care & Evaluate) 124
Active listening 25
Activities 144-155
   Craft 150
   Music 150
   Physical 150
   Recreational 150
   Relaxation 151
   Social group 151
   Spiritual 151
Activities of Daily Living (ADL) 13 16
Adaptations in the home 121
Aggression 164
Alcohol hand rub 51 53 55
Anxiety 32 145 146
Appetite 146 169
Assist Ireland 20

Bacteria 55 160
Balanced diet 5 79
Bed bath 14 60 61 63
Bereavement 23
Blood clots 146
Blood pressure 82 87 147 169 172
Body fluids 48 54 60 139 140 141 160 166

Body language 24 26 28 29 34 164
Bowel habits 169
Breathing difficulties 147

Cardiovascular system 145
Care equipment 98 135 136
Care plan 17 46 90 95 100 106 110 114 116 125
Challenging behaviour 163 164 165
Charts
   ABC Chart 165 166 172 186
   Bristol Stool Chart 106 107
   Falls Risk Assessment Chart 123 172 185
   Fluid balance chart 96 106 171 180
   Food Intake chart 179
   Mood chart 172 184
   Nutritional Assessment chart 179 187
   Observation chart 183
   Turns chart 132 133 172 182
   Waterlow Chart 131 134 171 181
Chest infections 147
Citizens information board 20
Cleanliness 135
Client documentation 168 170 171
Cognitive difficulties 32

INDEX

Cognitive activities 150
Cognitive benefits 145 146
Cognitive changes 169
Cognitive decline 147
Communication 5 13 20 24-35 40 45 109 112 121 150 151 164 168 175 176
  Active listening 24 25
  Barriers to communication 24 32
  Body Language 24 26 28 29 33 164
  Communication tips 30
  Eye contact 25 29 33 40
  Facial expressions 26 27 33 39 40
  Hearing problems 32 33
  Listening Skills 24 25
  Passive Listening 24
  Touch 27 29 176
  Verbal communication 26
  Visual aids 29 30
Concentration 146 150
Confidence 72 112 118 123 147 149
Confidentiality 24 27 32 46
Confrontation 164 165
Consent 31 39 56 61 63 71 91 100 110 115 116 133 144 148 156 157
Consultation 46 123 124
Contamination 48 55 94 136 137 139 140
Continence 98 103 104
Continuity of care 34 170
Culture 66 148 153
Cultural considerations -
  Continence Promotion 98 106

Grooming 69 75
Hygiene 45 66 67
Nutritional Needs 96
Social Activities 144 153
Cultural needs 66 175 177

Daily living aids 20
Data protection 46
De-escalation techniques 164
Dementia 20 23 163
Depression 23 145 146 178
Diet 5 79 80 96
  Dietitian 20 133
  Digestion 146
  Eating and drinking habits 169
  Malnutrition 20 21
Dignity 5 8 10 12 36 38 45 46 58 60 67 76 79 91 98 99 102 105 109 121 133 146
Disorientation 147
Doctor 17 27 38
Dress code 45 47 137
Dressing aids 77

Elisabeth Kubler Ross 178
  Loss and grief 175 177
Emotional needs 6
Empathy 5 10 28 36 40
End of life care 175
#endpjparalysis 76
Environmental needs 11
Ergonomic conditions 122 161

Falls Risk 125 172
Falls risk assessment 123 185
Family care 175 177
Fitness 145
Five stages of grief 175 177 178

Food pyramid 80
   Carbohydrates 81
   Proteins 81 95
   Fats 81 82 94
   Vitamins 81 82 83 85 95
   Minerals 81 83 86 95
   Water 81
Foul/infected linen 139 140
Friendships 145
Functional mobility 19

Grooming 45 58 69 70 71 75 155
   Hair 69 71-72 74 75 154
   Teeth 69 72 73 74 86 87 154
   Oral care 73 176
   Shaving 69 74
   Make-up 42 69 75
   Hand/foot care 54 74

Hand hygiene 45 47 49 50 51 53 55
   Alcohol rub 51 53 55
   Handwashing 50 53 55 62
Hazardous waste 141 159
Hazards 49 159 162
   Physical 159
   Chemical 160
   Biological 160
   Human factors 160
Health Act 2007 4
Hearing problems 32 33
Heart 18 82 83
'Hello my name is..' 38
HIQA 3 4 12
Holistic care 1 5
HSE Minimal Handling Policy 123
Hygiene standards 46 47 104

Immune system 81 85 88 145 146
Incontinence 98 99 103 139 141
   Incontinence pads 99 103
   Catheter care 104
   Stoma care 105
Injuries 18 22 116 123 147 169
Intellectual disability 3 29 163
Intergenerational projects 153
Isolation 5 146 147

Joints 19 89 146

Laundry 66 135 138-140
   Foul/infected linen 139 140
   Blue laundry bag 140
   Green laundry bag 140
   Red/Orange alginate bag 139
   Red laundry bag 139 140
   White laundry bag 139
   Yellow bin bags 141
Linen 138

Malnutrition 20 21
Mandatory training 165
Manual handling 109 110 111 112 122 123 132 156 158 159 160-162 165
Manual handling aids 109 111 112 161
   Bed rope ladder 113
   Bed rail 112
   Over-bed grab rail 113
   Sliding sheet 114
   PAT slide 114
   Banana board 114
Manual handling regulations 122
Maslow's Hierarchy of Needs 7-8

INDEX

Mechanical aids 115 118
   Hoist 58 63 64 100 118
Medical gases 160
Memory 25 146 150
Mental health needs 3 18 22
Mental illness 3 163
Mobility 19 20 109-126 131 145 147 150
Mobility aids 20 109 118 121 123
Mood 19 79 146 169 172 184
Motivation 6 77
Multidisciplinary team 16
Multiple sclerosis 18
Muscle function 18
Muscle strength 85 121 145
Musculoskeletal system 18 160

Negotiate 165
Nurses 16 17 76 168
Nutritional needs 79 90 175 176

Occupational therapist 19 70 78
Oral/history projects 153
Orthoptists 16 21

Pain management 175 176
Pain scores 172
Palliative care 178
Parkinson's disease 18
Pathogens 141 160
Personal hygiene 45 104 166
Personal space 28 39 43
Person-centred 11 12 67
Physical ailments 147
Physical disability 3
Physical needs 5 6 9 11 17 144
Physiotherapists 16 18 19
Podiatrist 16 22

Positive self-image 36 42 75 78
Personal Protective Equipment (PPE) 45 48 136
Pressure mattress 113 133
Pressure sores 113 127 128 129 131 132 134 147 175 176
Pressure sores risk assessment 134 171
Promoting Continence 98 103
   Incontinence aids 103 104 105
   Toileting aids 100-102
Psychiatrist 16 22
Psychological needs 5 6 7 10
Pulmonary disease 18

Reduced vision 21
Reminiscence 150
Reporting 106 138 168
Respect 79 109
Risk assessment 49 57 113 134 159 160 171 172
Roper, Logan & Tierney 13

Safety 158-167
Safety statement 158 159
Safety, Health & Welfare at Work Act 2005 158 159
Self-actualisation 6 7
Self-Esteem 8 61 72 118 147
Self-expression 146
Sensory equipment 69 70
   Sight 70
   Hearing 70
Sharps 139 142
Short-tempered 147
Sleeping pattern 169
Social needs 6 8 45 144
Socialisation 145

Special dietary requirements 93
　Modified textured diet 93
　Diabetes 94
　Coeliac disease 94
　Lactose intolerance 95
　Nut allergy 95
　Cystic fibrosis 94
　Vegetarianism 95
　Veganism 95
Special/additional needs 2 22
Speech & language therapy 16
Spillages 90 92 142 163
Spiritual needs 5 11 148
Staff immunisation 166
Stereotypes 147
Sterilising agents 160
Stress 6 22 145 160
Supervisor 25 31 32 67 75 90 95
　　96 100 106 110 114 116 125 134
Sympathy 5 40

30 degree tilt 132
TILE 161
Toileting aids 99-102
　Commode 98 99 100 101 102
　　104 105 115 136 137
　Bedpan 98 99 100 101 102 195
　　136
　Urinal 98 99 101 102 136
Transfer from bed to chair 114
Transfer in the bed 112

Urinary infections 146
Urinary output 169

Values in action 36 37
Verbal communication 24 26
Virus 160
Visual aids 29 30
Visual changes 169

Walking aids 111
　Walking sticks 118
　Quad walking sticks 119
　Walker/Zimmer frame 119
Warning cues 164
Washing aids 58
　Bed bath 9 60-63
　Assisted wash 9 60 63
Waste disposal 141
Waste Management 141
　Infectious waste 141
Weight loss/gain 131 169
Well-being 11 18 19 79 146 151
Wheelchair 20 99 109 110 114 115
　　119-120
World Health Organisation (WHO)
　　11

Acknowledgements:

To Finn and to Helen.
To all my friends and colleagues in the Childcare and Healthcare Department in Limerick College of Further Education, with special thanks to Blathnaid O'Donghue for her assistance and advice.
To all the students that have taught me so much.